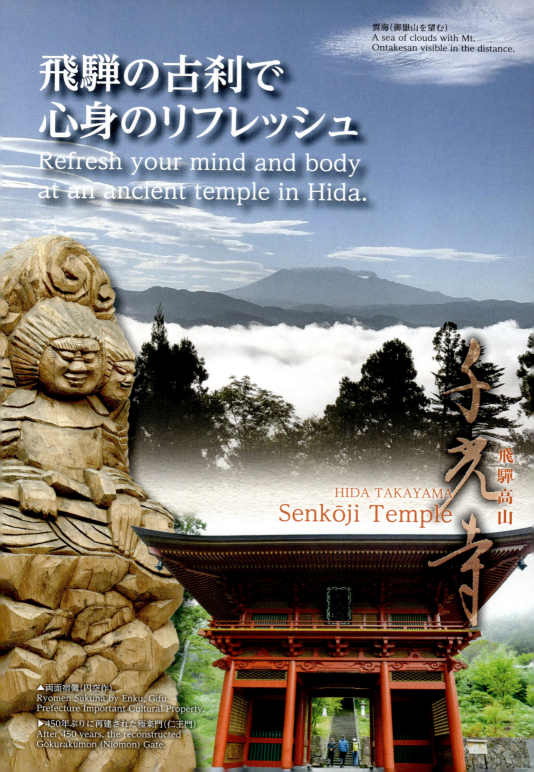

雲海（御嶽山を望む）
A sea of clouds with Mt. Ontakesan visible in the distance.

飛騨の古刹で心身のリフレッシュ
Refresh your mind and body at an ancient temple in Hida.

飛騨高山
HIDA TAKAYAMA
Senkōji Temple

▲ 両面宿儺（円空作）
Ryomen Sukuna by Enku, Gifu Prefecture Important Cultural Property.

▶ 450年ぶりに再建された極楽門（仁王門）
After 450 years, the reconstructed Gokurakumon (Niomon) Gate.

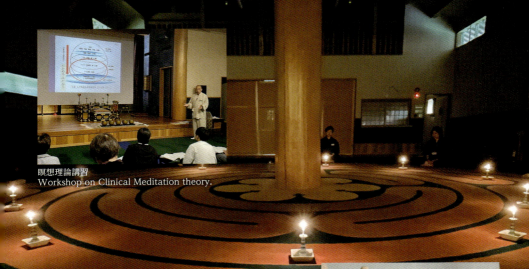

瞑想理論講習
Workshop on Clinical Meditation theory.

ラビリンスでたかめる瞑想の風景
Energizing meditation around the Labyrinth in the International Peace Meditation Center.

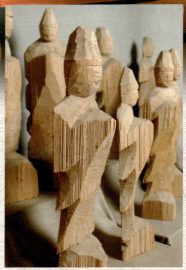

三十三観音（円空作）
33 Kannon (Avalokitesvara) Statues by Enku.

　飛騨国千光寺は、古え薫る仁徳天皇の御代、今から1600年前に飛騨の豪族 両面宿儺が古代信仰の祈りの場所として開き、約1200年前に真如法親王（弘法大師の十大弟子の1人）が仏教寺院として建立された古刹です。隆盛期には山上に19の伽藍、院坊が立ち並んでいましたが、永禄7年（1564）に甲斐の武田軍の飛騨攻めの際に兵火にかかり、一山全て炎上しました。のち天正16年（1588）に飛騨高山城主金森長近が名刹を偲んで再建したのが、現在の堂宇です。現在は高野山真言宗に属する密教寺院で、山岳仏教の修行の古風を今に伝えています。最近では「円空仏の寺」としても、その名は広く知られています。

　どうぞゆっくりと参拝し、山のエネルギーや空気、森林の生命力自体を感じてください。

円空図（県重要文化財）
Portrait of Enku, pigment and ink on Paper, Gifu Prefecture Important Cultural Property.

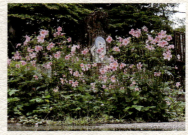

秋明菊
Shumeigiku-Japanese Anemone Flowers.

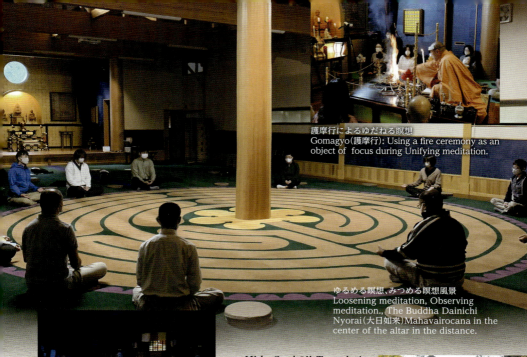

護摩行によるゆだねる瞑想
Gomagyo (護摩行): Using a fire ceremony as an object of focus during Unifying meditation.

ゆるめる瞑想、みつめる瞑想風景
Loosening meditation, Observing meditation., The Buddha Dainichi Nyorai (大日如来) Mahavairocana in the center of the altar in the distance.

千光寺本堂夜景
Night view of Senkōji, Temple Main Hall.

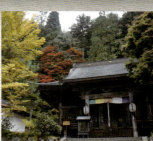

千光寺本堂
The grounds of Hida-Senkōji Temple.

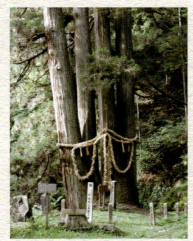

国の天然記念物「五本杉」
A Japanese cedar tree with five trunks from a single root.

Hida-Senkōji Temple is located in the mountains at 900 meters/3000 feet above sea level in central Japan. It was founded on the land said to be established as sacred grounds by Ryōmen-sukuna (両面宿儺) the head of a powerful clan family in Hida Province 1600 years ago during the reign of Emperor Nintoku (313–399 CE). Shinnyobō Shinnō (真如法親王), one of the ten great disciples of Kōbō Daishi, (774-835 CE) the founder of Esoteric Buddhism in Japan, established this temple 1200 years ago. Hida-Senkōji is an esoteric Buddhist temple belonging to the Kōyasan-Shingon Lineage and carried a long tradition of mountin asceticism.

The whole mountain is the subject of faith. When you have the opportunity, please enjoy a tranquil visit, to Hida Senkōji, feel the energy of the mountain, its fresh air, and the vitality of its forested landscape.

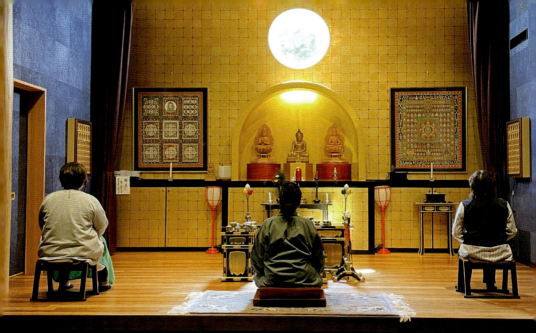

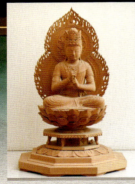

瞑想センターセンター本尊大日如来
The principal Buddhist image of Dainichi nyorai（大日如来）Mahavairocana Buddha.

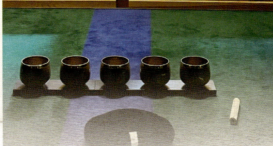

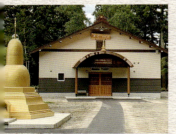

国際平和瞑想センターと仏舎利塔
Rear: International Peace Meditation Center, Front: Buddhist Relic Stupa.

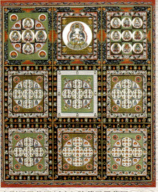

金剛界曼荼羅（左）と胎蔵界曼荼羅
Shingon Buddism's Mandala of the Two Realms, Diamond Realm (left) and Womb Realm (right).

セラピストのためのガイドブック

臨床瞑想法の メソッド紹介
～その魅力と実践法～ 【和文英文併記】

Introduction to the Clinical Meditation Method
It's Merits and a Practical Guide for Therapists and Care Providers
The Clinical Meditation Research Institute

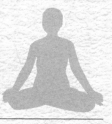

編著
臨床瞑想法教育研究所
大下大圓

Author's name
Ven. Daien Oshita
Ms. Keiko Miyamoto
Dr. Etsuyo Nishigaki
Dr. Hirohisa Saitō
Rev. Dr. Nathan Jishin Michon
Rev. Acharyā Ekō Noble

◉目次

はじめに　4

第1章　臨床瞑想法とは　12
１）今なぜ瞑想か…………12
２）臨床瞑想法の4つの瞑想メソッド…………14

第2章　実習編～事前準備　26
１）瞑想するための準備…………26
２）瞑想の開始…………32
３）内面への気づき…………42

第3章　4つの瞑想メソッド（実習に向けての理解）　50
１）ゆるめる瞑想法（緩和、集中型瞑想法）…………50
２）みつめる瞑想法（観察、洞察瞑想法）…………54
３）たかめる瞑想（生成、促進瞑想法）…………68
４）ゆだねる瞑想法（統合、融合瞑想法）…………78

第4章　対人援助のための臨床瞑想法のトレーニング　88
１）実施手順…………88
２）健常者を対象とするとき…………92
３）ベッドで療養されている方への臨床瞑想法…………98
４）臨床瞑想法に役立つ音楽の利用など…………104
５）臨床瞑想法実践のポイント…………106

第5章　臨床瞑想法指導者養成研修会の様子　110

◉Contents

Forward　5

Section 1　Defining the Clinical Meditation Method　13

1) The importance of meditation in today's world⋯⋯⋯⋯13

2) Four types of Clinical Meditation⋯⋯⋯⋯17

Section 2　Meditation　27

1) Preparing for meditation⋯⋯⋯⋯27

2) Beginning meditation⋯⋯⋯⋯33

3) Awareness of the inner mind⋯⋯⋯⋯43

Section 3　Four methods of meditation
（Preparing for meditation practice）　51

1) "Loosening Meditation" (relief/concentration)⋯⋯⋯⋯51

2) "Observing Meditation" (watching/insight)⋯⋯⋯⋯55

3) "Energizing Meditation" (creation/reverence)⋯⋯⋯⋯71

4) "Unifying Meditation" (integration/unification)⋯⋯⋯⋯81

Section 4　How Clinical Meditation for Interpersonal Support is practiced in the Japanese Cultural Context　89

1) Implementation procedures⋯⋯⋯⋯89

2) When targeting healthy individuals⋯⋯⋯⋯93

3) Clinical Meditation for Clients who are sick in bed⋯⋯⋯⋯99

4) Using Music with Clinical Meditation⋯⋯⋯⋯103

5) The keys for practicing Clinical Meditation⋯⋯⋯⋯105

Section 5　Certificate program for leaders of Clinical Meditation　111

Afterword　119

はじめに

　本書は、臨床瞑想法教育研究所で考案した「臨床瞑想法」の解説書です。

　考案者であり本書の編者代表の大下大圓（臨床瞑想法教育研究所代表）は、高野山（仏教、真言密教の本山）やスリランカ（初期仏教を代表とするテーラヴァーダーの教え）で瞑想修行の後に、京都大学こころの未来研究センターで瞑想の臨床応用を研究し「臨床瞑想法」を考案しました。京都大学では、世界の瞑想についての先行研究を精査し、それぞれの瞑想のもつ機能性や目的、活用法や、現代の医科学や心理学などの知見および仏教瞑想の特性を吟味し、それらの統合化をはかりました。

　その背景について簡単に説明をしますと、編者大下は 12 歳で古刹飛騨千光寺において仏門出家し、高野山やスリランカで仏教・密教修行のなかで瞑想を習得しました。瞑想は伝統仏教において、あらゆる修行生活の要に応用されており、心身の鍛錬やスピリチュアリティの向上に有用な技法を保持しています。瞑想には多くの機能性がありながらも、これまで仏教界内部では宗派内の僧侶や信徒のみに温存され、外部に広く普及することはありませんでした。

　編者は専門的仏教修行を終えたのちに、医療や福祉の現場で患者・家族のセラピーにこれまで 40 年近く関わっていますが、その過程で瞑想を療法（セラピー）として活用するようになり、患者さんや家族、そしてケアする側の人たちにもその有用性を確認した手ごたえから、臨床応用できるものと確信しました。

　しかし、当時の医療現場では瞑想の応用や方法などは確立しておらず、手探りが続きました。特に日本の公共空間においては、宗教的作法の行使には難しい現実的課題がありました。代替療法の観点からヨーガ療法は少しずつ採用されているときでした。

　そんな折にアメリカからマインドフルネス瞑想が入ってきました。それ

Forward

Although Buddhist meditation has many pragmatic and useful applications, it was long known only to Buddhist priests and lay practitioners. It took time to begin spreading outside the walls and confines of temples and those who practiced there. Yet for me, this broader teaching and application of such meditation skills has become one of my greatest life passions and projects.

When only twelve years old I decided to become a Buddhist priest at Hida Senkōji, a remote yet beautiful and historic temple in the mountains of central Japan. It is a temple from the Shingon tradition, a form of Esoteric Buddhism with many types of meditation. Meditation and meditative practices are key in all aspects of training in traditional Buddhism as they help one to acquire useful skills for training the body and the mind as well as enhancing spirituality. I deepened my practice of meditation during my Buddhist training in Kōyasan, the sacred mountain town south of Osaka, which is the center of Shingon practice. Then I decided to learn other practices maintained in the Theravada lineage of Early Buddhism in Sri Lanka. After I completed my various priestly trainings in Buddhism, I became a licensed music therapist, helping patients and their family members in medical and welfare settings and I am a Certified Therapist of the Japan Holistic Medical Association. I found my background in meditation practices to actually be very applicable and helpful for many of the people in such clinical settings. At that time, the therapeutic use of meditation was not yet established in such medical settings. Furthermore, religious-based practices were not readily accepted in public spaces in Japan back then. Around the same time, yoga therapy

は宗教性を排除した瞑想法であることから、医療や学校で使用されるようになりました。しかし、私がそれまでに習得した瞑想に照らしてみて、そのマインドフルネス瞑想だけでは満足できるものを与えてはくれませんでした。臨床瞑想法の「たかめる瞑想」「ゆだねる瞑想」はセラピーでは大事な部分を構成しますが、その部分がマインドフルネスにはあまり採用されていません。

　そこで、日本人の心情や宗教性を考慮し、臨床場面でも活用可能な瞑想法の確立が必要となったのです。それが京都大学でのメソッド開発につながりました。

　日本の公共空間では、宗教性を用いない瞑想が受け入れられやすい傾向にあります。臨床瞑想法はそういったことを考慮して、あらたな使命と役割を担うこととなりました。それはマインドフルネス瞑想が不要という評価ではなく、瞑想療法にはもっと多様性があり、マインドフルネス瞑想を補完するものになると考えました。

　臨床瞑想法は、編者が仏教の僧侶であることから伝統的に活用されていた仏教瞑想が基本になって考案したものですが、この臨床瞑想法は、「宗教性を用いなくても実践できる」ように工夫されています。瞑想の基礎から順番に段階的に瞑想法を学ぶことで、より深い瞑想の境地を体験することができます。従ってこの臨床瞑想法には、非宗教的側面からでも、あるいは宗教性を用いても実施できるという２つの利用法が可能となっているのです。

　また瞑想する人が精神的な支えとして、宗教（仏教、キリスト教、イスラム教など）を信奉している場合は、その宗教心理を内面に保持しつつ、臨床瞑想法を実施することができます。例えば、特に仏教的な背景を持つ人は「みつめる瞑想、たかめる瞑想」で、その人自身の洞察的な要素や健康恢復へのアプローチに、仏教の要素を加味することが可能です。同様に他の宗教でも、その宗教がもっている強み——例えば人間性や霊性の向上に関する内容——を「たかめる瞑想」のところで引用し、工夫して活用することも可能です。とくに「ゆだねる瞑想」ではそれぞれの宗教性の特徴的な祈りを反映して「臨床瞑想法」を実施することもできます。ただし、援助として行う瞑想で宗教

began to be accepted as an alternative therapy little by little, and the secularized clinical aspects of mindfulness meditation were imported from the USA. Mindfulness meditation was accepted easily in medical settings and schools because it excluded religiosity. However, I found mindfulness meditation alone unsatisfactory in light of what I learned from various methods of meditation. I do not mean to say that mindfulness meditation is unnecessary, but that there are other kinds of meditation conducive to clinical applications capable of complementing mindfulness meditation. That is, the western secular forms of mindfulness practice do not include "Energizing Meditation" and "Unifying Meditation," which play important therapeutic roles in the Clinical Meditation Method. These circumstances provided the Clinical Meditation Method with a new mission and role. I explored clinical applications of meditation therapy at Kyoto University's Kokoro Research Center: I investigated previous works about meditation around the world, categorized the functions, usages, and goals of meditation across regions and religions. Then, I integrated the products of my investigation, knowledge of Buddhism, and information of modern medicine and psychology. The result is the "Clinical Meditation Method." I hoped that establishing a new form of meditation for clinical settings would consider the sentiments and religiosity of the Japanese. Yet, I believe the resulting method is applicable far beyond the borders of Japan. I have now provided meditation as a part of therapy for about forty years and these decades of experience helped convince me that this method of Clinical Meditation is very useful not only for clients and their family members, but also for professional caregivers.

Public spaces in Japan tend to accept only secular forms of meditation.

This method is based on Buddhist meditation because I am a Buddhist priest. However, it is devised in such a way that anyone can practice it without necessarily being Buddhist or religious. Everybody can experience

性を活用する場合には、事前に瞑想参加者の同意を得ておくこともセラピスト（瞑想リーダー）として心得ておくポイントです。

この臨床瞑想法の開始後約 10 年間にわたって日本の医師、看護師などを中心に、瞑想実践を積み重ねて臨床に応用できるか否かを検討した実績があります。また近年には、日本学術振興会の研究として臨床瞑想法が採択され、現在「認知症患者や家族への瞑想応用」の研究を実施中です。他には「災害被災地での瞑想療法」、「企業人のメンタルヘルスを図る瞑想活用」や「軽度認知機能障害や認知症者の介護者のストレス軽減の研究」などを実施し、生理学的、心理精神医学的エビデンスを獲得してきました。[1]

ここに自信をもって、世界にアピールできる瞑想法を紹介させていただきます。

本書は「臨床瞑想法」の簡単な理論と実習とで構成されています。

まずは入門的な臨床瞑想法の理解と、つぎに実践編を紹介して、瞑想経験者であればすぐに応用できるように紹介しています。

実習編の特徴は、自らの瞑想を深める方法（自利）と他者に応用する（利他）臨床瞑想法の 2 つの手順を示します。自分のための瞑想を深めつつ、対人援助としての瞑想法でもあります。

したがって、本書は誰にも応用できる瞑想の入門的ガイドブックでありつつ、特に医療、福祉、介護、教育などの対人援助の分野で、ケア者自身のスピリチュアリティの向上に役立つだけでなく、人のストレス軽減などの予防医学的な視点などでの活用も可能となっています。

本書の製作には、構成、翻訳、研究協力などでお世話になった方が沢山いますが、あとがきで紹介させていただきます。

本書をテキストとして活用し、臨床瞑想法の理解と実践の拡大によって、人々と世界のこころの平安に貢献できたならば、それは編者のもっとも希望とするところであります。

また本書の資料としては、多くは編者の著作から引用しています。

『即身成仏観法入門』青山社、2021

deep and advanced meditation by learning the basics of this method, step by step.

If a meditator believes in a religion (e.g., Buddhism, Christianity, Islam, etc.) as his or her spiritual support, they can use this method while still internally maintaining their religious principles. However, when the therapist leads a meditation, it is imperative for him or her to obtain participants' consent before incorporating religiosity into the method.

I repeatedly practiced this method with physicians, nurses, and other health professionals for the first ten years to examine the viability of its clinical application. Recently, my collaborators and I also obtained a Grant-in-Aid for Scientific Research from the Japan Society for the Promotion of Science, part of the Japanese Ministry of Education, Culture, Sports, Science and Technology [MEXT] for our new research project, "The practice of meditation for dementia patients and their family members." Our other research projects, to date, obtaining physiological and psychological evidence include, "The use of meditation for office workers to lower stress" and "Meditation for lowering stress among caregivers of patients with mild cognitive impairment or dementia".[1] So, encouraged by the results of this research, I present the Clinical Meditation Method which I confidently believe could be useful for anyone in the world.

This book consists of two main parts: basic theory and practice.

First, I present the basics of the Clinical Meditation Method, and then illustrate how the method is practiced. For those who have previously practiced meditation, this method can be used immediately. In presenting the Practice, I show two procedures to deepen meditation for oneself (自利 Jiri) and to altruistically share your practice with others (利他 Rita). That is, you can enhance yourself by learning and practicing while you also hold the aspiration to benefit others with this method.

In short, this book is an introductory guide and textbook that can

『ACP 人生会議でこころのケア』ビィング・ネット・プレス、2020
『瞑想力』日本評論社、2019
『臨床瞑想法』日本看護協会出版会、2016
『実践的スピリチュアルケア』日本看護協会出版会、2014
『瞑想療法』医学書院、2010

be used not only for enhancing one's sense of spirituality in the role of a caregiver in various fields of interpersonal assistance, such as medicine, welfare, care, and education, but also for lowering stress, improving health, and potentially preventing illness among one's colleagues.

Many people helped me with the composition, translation, research, and other aspects of this book. I acknowledge their help in the Afterword.

I hope this book will contribute to peace of mind among people all over the world by spreading the theory and practice of Clinical Meditation.

This book draws on my previous works in Japanese as follows:

大下大圓 Oshita Daien. (2021). *即身成仏観法入門 Sokushin jōbutsu kanpō nyūmon*, 青山社 Seizan sha.

大下大圓 Oshita Daien. (2020). *ACP 人生会議で心のケア ACP Jinsei kaigi de kokoro no kea*, ビィングネットプレス Biing net presu.

大下大圓 Oshita Daien. (2019). *瞑想力 Meisō ryoku*, 日本評論社 Nihon hyōron sha.

大下大圓 Oshita Daien. (2010). *瞑想療法 Meisō ryōhō*, 医学書院 Igaku sho in.

大下大圓 Oshita Daien. (2014). *実践的スピリチュアルケア Jissennteki spiricharu kea*, 日本看護協会出版会 Nihon kango kyōkai shuppan kai.

第1章

臨床瞑想法とは

1）今なぜ瞑想か

現代はストレス社会といわれています。

一般にストレスは、自律神経やホルモン系、免疫系に影響がでて、イライラ感、不安感、憂うつ気分、悲しみなどの心理面や、身体面では、動悸、だるさ、息苦しさ、口渇、冷や汗などの症状で表されます。そのときには反応として、アルコール類・タバコに頼ったり、職場でのミスも増えたり、遅刻するなどの影響がでてしまいます。

しかし、ストレスの全てが悪いものではありません。ストレスはユーストレス（ポジティブ要因）という考え方もあって、適度な刺激や超えるべき壁として、自身を高める方向に活用することもできるのです。瞑想を活用することで、ディストレス（ネガティブ要因）をユーストレスに変容する可能性があるのです。

日本成人病予防協会では、ユーストレスは「快い適度の刺激」「目標」と言いかえてもよく、適度のストレスは、意欲や向上心を掻き立て、イキイキとした張りのある生活のためには必要なものとしています。逆にディストレスは「過度の刺激」「プレッシャー」と言いかえることができ、親しい人の死やリストラにあって職を失うといった強い情動は、意欲を停滞させやがては健康を損なってしまうと説明しています。[2]

つまりこの臨床瞑想法を実施することで、①ストレスを解放するために「心をゆるめて、今の自分を知ること」が可能になり、その後②ストレス状態からの回復促進として「自心の修復から、あらたな未来へ」気持ちを切り替えられることが期待されます。

12●第1章　臨床瞑想法とは

Section 1.

Defining the Clinical Meditation Method

1) The importance of meditation in today's world

Modern society has many stressors. Generally, stress negatively affects autonomic nervous, endocrine, and immune systems, causing psychological responses like irritation, anxiety, depression, and grief, as well as physical responses like heart palpitations, fatigue, dyspnea, dry mouth, and cold sweats. This can lead people toward drinking or smoking, arriving late to work, or making more errors in the workplace.

However, stress is not always bad. Stress can be seen as a positive factor called "eustress" that enhances one's life through appropriate stimulation. In fact, meditation makes it possible to transform distress (a negative factor) into eustress.

The Japan Association of Preventive Medicine for Adult Diseases explains that eustress can be an "appropriate stimulus" and "challenge," which motivates people to live actively and pursue their inspirations, whereas distress can be an "excessive stimulus" and "pressure," and strong emotions triggered by the loss of a loved one or a job tends to lower motivation and negatively affect health.[2]

Here, the Clinical Meditation Method is expected to help people ① release their stress by "relaxing and knowing themselves in the present moment" and ② recover from stressful conditions by "restoring their minds and orienting them to new futures."

Take a balloon for example. When pressed by a hand (a stressor),

風船の動きで例えると、本来丸い風船（心）を上から手（ストレッサー）で押さえると変形しますね。これがストレスのかかった心を表します。でも、その手を放すと元の丸い風船に戻ります。これが回復です。風船を押す力は同じでも、よく膨らんだ風船はすぐに回復します。瞑想によって、心のレジリエンスが増し、ストレッサーもユーストレスになるのです。こんな風にこころを多面的にみてゆくことができる作業が瞑想でもあります。

　「瞑想」は、実は紀元前13世紀のインド最古の聖典『リグ＝ヴェーダ』には、すでに洗練された瞑想法があったようです。古代インダス文明の遺跡から出土した坐像印章には、瞑想するシヴァ神とも解釈できるデザインのものが発見されていることからも、瞑想は人類悠久の自己省察のツールといえます。

　瞑想は、伝統宗教の仏教やキリスト教などにおいては心身の鍛錬に活用されてきました。古代インドのバラモンらによる「瞑想ヨーガ」や、仏教において中心的な修行である「禅定・瞑想」は、宗教的には人間育成の重要なトレーニングでした。

　近年において瞑想は特定の民族、宗教や地域に偏ることなく、前出のように人のストレスを軽減し、心身の機能を高め、精神安定や健康増進に有効であることが多くの臨床研究から明らかにされてきました。

　そして今や瞑想は、世界のあらゆる場所や空間でひろく活用されており、医学や教育の場にも導入されて、人格育成や予防医学、代替療法、健康生成のプログラムとして活用されているのです。

　瞑想（meditation）とは「静かに自心を省察し、内なる声に耳を澄ますこと」です。その目的とするところを『心理療法事典』では「弛緩の促進、ストレス緩和の援助、自尊心を高めること、集中力の促進、現在中心の意識の発達、洞察の促進」（1999、青土社）と記されています。このことからも、瞑想には多義的な解釈や方法、目的があることがわかります。

２）臨床瞑想法の4つの瞑想メソッド

　本書が提示する「臨床瞑想法」の「4つのメソッド」を概説します。

a round-shaped balloon (a mind) gets deformed (stressed). When the hand is removed, however, the balloon returns to its original shape. This is recovery. Controlling for the pressure from the hand, a better inflated balloon recovers its original shape more quickly. With the help of meditation, one's mind becomes more resilient, and a stressor becomes eustress. Meditation thus reveals the multidimensional nature of the mind.

The Rig-Veda, among the world's oldest sacred texts dating back to 1300 BC in India, indicates that a sophisticated method of meditation was already established at that time. A carved depiction of a meditating Indian deity, Shiva, was unearthed from the ruins of the ancient Indus Valley civilization, so meditation can be seen as humanity's ancient tool for self-reflection.

Meditation has been used for training the mind and body in traditional religions, such as Buddhism and Christianity. "Meditation Yoga" in Brahmanism and "禅定 Zenjō," deeply concentrated meditation in Buddhism, are essential to their respective ascetic practices, and have served as important vehicles of human development. Moreover, many clinical studies in recent years show that meditation lowers stress, improves brain and physical functioning, and helps stabilize and enhance mental health irrespective of race, region or religion. Meditation is now widely practiced around the world, introduced into the fields of medicine and education, and used as programs for character building, preventative medicine, alternative therapy, and health promotion.

In essence, meditation is "an act of calmly examining one's own mind and listening to one's internal voice." According to *The Psychotherapy Encyclopedia* (1999. 青土社), the aim of meditation is "to promote relaxation, help lower stress, improve dignity, enhance concentration, develop consciousness centered upon the present moment, and deepen insight." This indicates that meditation has many meanings, methods, and goals.

● 「ゆるめる瞑想」

「ゆるめる瞑想」は、心身の緩和と集中を目的としています。緩和するために、意図的（恣意的）に呼吸と身体のリズムを調和させます。

たとえば、忙しいあなたが、一日の仕事が終わって、お風呂に入るとどんな気持ちになりますか？　ゆったりとした気分になれますよね。このまったりした気持ちを瞑想で味わうのが、「ゆるめる瞑想」なのです。

普段、呼吸は無意識に行っていますが、「ゆるめる瞑想」中は、意識的に呼吸を行います。意識する呼吸とは、息を吐くことを意識的に長く行うことで、副交感神経を優位に導き、脳波をアルファ波状態にすることよって、セロトニン神経の働きでエンドルフィンなどの脳内神経伝達物質の分泌を促すのです。たとえ緊張状態で交感神経が優位になり、ベータ波の状態であっても、そこから深い呼吸と意図的な呼吸をコントロールすることによって、脳波や自律神経に働きかけて、緊張から心身の弛緩状態を醸し出すことができるというのがゆるめる瞑想なのです。

緩和された意識は次第に集中した意識状態を醸し出し、次の「みつめる瞑想」に移行します。集中意識は呼吸の動きに注視することで達成されていきます。

● 「みつめる瞑想」

「みつめる瞑想」は、観察することと洞察することです。十分な緩和によって得られた集中的な意識状態は、自己や他者を客観的に観察することのできる冷静な心の状態になります。そのままの自分をみることが観察です。観察とは文字どおり、自我意識にとらわれないで対象をどこまでも客観的に見続けることです。

それは注意に基づく瞑想であり、ものごとを客観的に、第三者的に観察し続けることです。最近は「マインドフルネス瞑想」というフレーズで有名ですが、もともとマインドフルネス（Mindfulness）とは、初期仏教のパーリ語の（Sati ＝念・正念）に由来するものとして、英訳されたものが日本にもた

2) Four types of Clinical Meditation

- **"Loosening Meditation"** (relaxation/concentration)

Loosening Meditation aims at relaxing the mind and body and increasing concentration. To loosen is to intentionally harmonize breath with the rhythm of the body. How do you feel when you soak in the bath, or take a hot shower after a busy day? You certainly feel comfortable, right? You can experience this relaxing feeling in "Loosening Meditation."

While you might not be aware of your breathing in your daily life, during "Loosening Meditation" you breathe consciously. An intentionally long outbreath activates the parasympathetic nervous system and generates alpha waves, triggering serotonin neurons to increase neurotransmitters like endorphins. Even when you are nervous and the sympathetic nervous system and beta waves in the brain are dominant, deep and conscious breathing through a Loosening Meditation shifts the brain waves and the autonomic nervous system in the direction of mental and physical relaxation. The relaxed mind eventually develops into a focused state of consciousness, transitioning into the next "Observing Meditation." Such focused consciousness is enabled by closely observing the rhythms of breathing.

- **"Observing Meditation"** (watching/insight)

"Observing Meditation" (watching/insight) refers to observing and gaining insight. Concentration, as the result of sufficient relaxation, lets you calmly observe yourself and others. Observation is, as the name suggests, an act of maintaining an objective awareness of the object without becoming self-conscious.

It is a meditation based on concentrated awareness that maintains an

らされました。

　一般には「Sati」は「気づき」などと解釈され、マインドフルネスでは「注意・観察」の意味になります。仏教では偏りを離れた中道の心で、ありのままに対象を観るという瞑想のことをいいます。そこでは、観察する主観的な自己と、観察される客観的な自己を見分けてみることも可能です。

　さらにそれが進むと洞察になります。洞察は分析と似ていますが、分析はどちらかというと、物事を細分化する二元論的な要素がありますが、洞察は常に全体を眺めつつ、その本質を深くほりさげる感覚です。例えば、ここにリンゴの実があります。まずそのリンゴの色や形を概観的に観察します。しかし中味がどうなっているかは、外からはわかりません。そこでもっと鼻を近づけて匂いを嗅いだり、一口かじってみたりして、味や硬さなどを知ります。この中味を知ったときが洞察です。

　これを自己の生育歴を洞察するときに応用すると、家族の関係性の全体像をみながら、そこで個人が対人とどのような関係であったか、思いを巡らし、どのような行動につながったかなどを、具体的に注意を凝らして深く見ていくような見方が洞察瞑想なのです。

　伝統仏教では四諦（苦・集・滅・道）と八正道（八聖道）（正しく見る、正しく思う、正しく語る、正しく命を運ぶ、正しく生業をする、正しく精進する、正しく念ずる、正しく定に入る）の洞察瞑想が、その究極の実践法として継承されてきました。

　八正道は「正見：ものごとを正しく見て理解すること、正思：正しい意図または目的、正語：虚偽を避け真実性を正しく語ること、正業：倫理に則った正しい行為、正命：正しく精神的な成長を目的とした生計、正精進：正しい努力によってポジティブな資質を培いネガティブな性質を克服する、正念：正しく記憶、自分の思考、感情、行動に気づき思念すること、正定：正しく集中力のある精神状態を向上すること」です。

- **「たかめる瞑想」**

「たかめる瞑想」は、心身の機能をアップさせようとする意識的なものです。

objective, third-person view. Lately the phrase "mindfulness meditation" is popular, and mindfulness originates from the Pali word "sati" in Early Buddhism. The Pali word was translated into English and then re-imported back into Japan (although Japanese does have an older, traditional word for mindfulness, Nen 念).

"Sati" generally means "awareness" and, in the context of mindfulness, "attention/observation." In Buddhism, "sati" meditation means an unbiased and neutral perspective on things as they really are. This Observing Meditation can differentiate the subjective, observing self and the objective, observed self.

This observation develops further into insight. Insight is similar to analysis but different. While analysis tends to divide an object into smaller components in a dualistic manner, insight means grasping an overall picture and penetrating deeply into the essence of an object. When you observe an apple, for example, you look at its color and shape, but you do not understand what is inside. So, you also smell, bite, and taste it. When you understand the inside of the apple, you gain insight. When applying this to your own upbringing and background, for example, you carefully and concretely examine your relationships and interactions with particular family members while looking at the totality of family relationships. This is "Observing Meditation."

In Buddhism, the insight meditation on the Four Noble Truths 四諦 (Suffering, Cause of Suffering, Cession of Suffering, Path to the Cession of Suffering) and Noble Eightfold Path 八聖道 (Right View, Right Intention, Right Speech, Right Action, Right Livelihood, Right Effort, Right Mindfulness, Right Concentration) has been inherited as the ultimate method.

Section 1.　Defining the Clinical Meditation Method●19

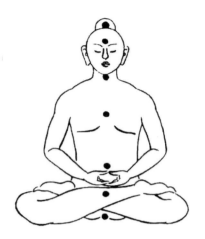

図1(fig.1) 瞑想とチャクラのイメージ（山崎泰廣、1970）
Meditation and Chakras

　この瞑想は人間の五官六根や五体の感覚や働きを意識しつつ、その機能性をより向上させていこうとする瞑想法です。
　たかめる瞑想は身体的側面と心理的側面の両面からアプローチしていきます。身体的には健康生成論に基づく健康増進や予防医学に基づく瞑想法です。[3]
　心理的には、1950年代以降に始まった人間性心理学に加えて、トランスパーソナル心理学の応用や、仏教、密教の修行法に多くのヒントや実践法があります。人のスピリチュアリティの向上が「たかめる瞑想」の目標となります。[4]
　特にヨーガや仏教（密教）では、人間の五体（下腹部、胃腸、心臓・肺、首・顔、頭頂）と宇宙のチャクラ（人体内のエネルギースポット）や五大要素、すなわち地水火風空の元素を同格とみて、それぞれのもつ機能を呼吸、身体運動、意識変容などで、現在よりもたかめていくことを目指します。（図1）それによって、生理学的にはホリスティック（全体的）に内分泌系、自律神経系、免疫系に働きかけて、それぞれの不調和な状態からバランスをとりつつ、部

正　見 (Right View) - Right understanding of the nature of existence
正　思 (Right Intention) - Right intention or purpose
正　語 (Right Speech) - Right speech, avoiding falsehood and promoting truthfulness
正　業 (Right Action) - Right conduct, following ethical principles
正　命 (Right Livelihood) - Right livelihood, earning a living in a way that is ethical and supports spiritual growth
正精進 (Right Effort) - Right effort, cultivating positive qualities and overcoming negative ones
正　念 (Right Mindfulness) - Right mindfulness, being aware of one's thoughts, feelings, and actions
正　定 (Right Concentration) - Right concentration, developing focused and concentrated mental states

- **"Energizing Meditation" (creation/reverence)**

"Energizing Meditation" (creation/reverence) is intended to enhance the functioning of the mind and body. This style of meditation cultivates awareness of the whole body and mind as well as the five senses, while improving their overall function.

Energizing Meditation includes both physical and psychological approaches. The physical approach is based on health promotion through salutogenesis as well as preventative medicine.[3] The psychological approach is based on humanistic psychology that started in the 1950s as well as derived from transpersonal psychology[4] and training methods in Early, non-Esoteric and Esoteric Buddhism. The aim of "Energizing Meditation" is to energize the body and mind in a deeper, almost spiritual way.

Yoga and Esoteric Buddhism traditionally conceptualize the five elements of the human body (lower abdomen, stomach, heart and lung, neck and face, top of the head) in accordance with five elements of the universe or "chakras" (energy spots in the human body), associated

Section 1.　Defining the Clinical Meditation Method●21

位によってはその機能向上をはかるものです。

　たとえば、家の中でくすぶっているよりは、カラオケに行って、自分の大好きな歌を思いっきり歌った方が、気分が上がるときもあります。実際に声を出して歌って身体に振動を与えることによって精神的な達成感が生じるという心身反応は、ドーパミンが神経に働きかけて脳内でドーパミンを分泌するからです。快楽物質が活性化することで気分の向上や肺活量などの機能が向上します。たかめる瞑想では、短いお経や真言（マントラ）を繰り返して、いったん意欲は高揚させますが、深い呼吸法でセロトニンが促され、落ち着きを取り戻し、その後に深い瞑想に入ることが可能となります。

● 「ゆだねる瞑想」

　「ゆだねる瞑想」は「たかめる瞑想」に連動して起きるものですから、その違いを明確に分けることは難しいものです。なぜなら、たかめる過程で、ゆだねる意識状態が出現することがあるからです。あえていえば「たかめる瞑想」は身体レベルの機能向上を目指しつつ、精神的な領域も次元上昇が出現し、連続して「ゆだねる」という感覚が心に生じて、おおらかな意識の状態に移行することです。これをトランスパーソナル心理学では変性意識といいます。これらの瞑想によって高次のスピリチュアリティが出現することを意味します。

　千光寺で臨床瞑想法を修練した女性は、このゆだねる瞑想で「自分の意識が拡大して宇宙に浮かんでいるような幸せな気分」を長時間にわたって味わったと言っていました。したがって、「ゆだねる瞑想」は自我意識を超克して、大いなる意識（サムシンググレイトなど）に融合、あるいは統合する意識状態といえます。

　宗教的な文脈では、神仏や天の領域につながることであり、仏教的には覚醒や悟りの状態に関連することを意味します。臨床瞑想法を習得することによって、誰もがこの境地を獲得できるということではなく、そういう目標がこの瞑想法の中にあるということです。

　ちょっと難しい表現かもしれませんが、これが瞑想の奥義ともいえる深い

with the elements of earth, water, fire, wind, and universe, respectively. (see fig.1) They aim at enhancing each function through breathwork, physical movements, and alterations of consciousness. Physiologically speaking, Energizing Meditation thus enables us to holistically activate the endocrine, autonomic nervous, and immune systems, dissolve their internal disharmony, and even enhance their functioning.

For example, your mood might improve when you go to sing your favorite songs at a Karaoke club instead of staying home and passing your time in idleness. Singing aloud vibrates the body and induces a sense of fulfilment in the mind because it stimulates dopamine neurons, triggering the brain to secrete that hormone. Secreting happiness hormones makes you feel refreshed and increases your lung capacity. In Energizing Meditation, you repeat short mantras or song-like phrases first, which temporarily makes you feel exalted, but deep breathing helps increase serotonin and regain calmness, leading into a deeper state of meditation.

- **"Unifying Meditation" (integration/entrusting)**

"Unifying Meditation" (integration/entrusting) can occur in conjunction with Energizing Meditation. It is difficult to strictly separate them because a unified state of consciousness can appear during the process of energizing the mind. Nevertheless, their difference can be stated as follows: "Energizing Meditation" enhances our physical functions and can heighten our sense of spirituality, which creates the feeling of Unification in the mind and consequently leads to an equanimous state of consciousness. In transpersonal psychology, this is called an altered state of consciousness. This means that some sense of a higher state of spirituality can emerge through energizing and unifying meditations.

A woman who practiced meditation at Hida Senkōji temple said that she enjoyed a feeling of happiness as if her sense of consciousness

世界です。ぜひあなたも瞑想であなた自身のこころの世界を探検してみましょう。

expanded and seemed to float in space for a long time. Unifying Meditation thus leads to a state of transcending ego-consciousness and a sense of merging or integrating with "Something Greater."

It is at this point that the beneficial experience of a unifying (entrusting) state transcending ego-conscious could be described and interpreted as religious experience, explained in terms of psychology, or using other philosophical systems. The Clinical Meditation Method, with its roots in Buddhism, offers the steps to this experience.

This may be difficult to describe, but it indicates a profound state within the heart of meditative experience. I encourage you to explore the world of your own mind through the meditative experience.

第2章

実習編～事前準備

1）瞑想するための準備

•身体のバランスを確認する

　まずは、身体の調整が必要です。いきなり「瞑想をやれ」といわれても戸惑うばかりだと思いますが、実は瞑想の前に確認しておくことがあります。スポーツをするときに必要な道具や準備体操をしてからでないと、思わぬ怪我をしてしまう。それと同じです。

　瞑想は坐るだけなので、そんなに準備はいりません。でもここに大きな落とし穴があります。坐るだけなのですが、ある程度の時間（5分以上）を同じ姿勢で保持するので、不自然な姿勢では心や体はかえって疲れてしまい、効果が損なわれます。そこで、瞑想を行うための最小限の心と身体の準備が必要となります。

•まずは環境を整える

　まずは瞑想を行う場所から考えましょう。

　基本的に瞑想は場所を選びません。本来は坐る場所さえあれば、どこでもできるのです。編者はよく旅行をしますが、移動で利用する飛行機や電車や列車、車の中で瞑想することがあります。また待合のイスや仕事の合間の時間などでも三昧（samadhi＝やすらかで平安な意識状態）に入ると、たとえ周りの騒音がうるさいところであっても、自己に集中することができます。しかしこれには少し訓練が必要です。

　初めて瞑想をやろうとする人は、やはり静かな環境を選ぶことをお奨めします。それは本当にどこでもいいのです。あなた自身のライフスタイルのな

Section 2.

Meditation

1) Preparing for meditation

• **Preparing physical conditions**

"Beginning meditation" may bewilder you. Of course, you do not necessarily start meditating out of the blue just like that! It is important that you prepare to meditate similar to preparing for sports or other activities. If not, the session simply might not go as well as it otherwise could.

This does not mean you are absolutely required to follow a long string of exact procedures. However, there are a number of physical, mental, and environmental preparations that can help provide better circumstances for your experience. For instance, sitting with a posture that is either too tight or too loose can impact your frame of mind. And if we go into any experience without expecting it to work, it probably won't work! Noticing our frame of mind and entering with the right attitude is also important.

• **Arrange your surroundings**

Where do you meditate? Basically, you can meditate anywhere you can sit. As I often travel, I meditate on airplanes, trains, and cars. I can focus my conscious attention on myself in a waiting room or during breaks despite loud background noise if I enter samadhi (a calm and peaceful) state of mind. Entering such a state of mind does take practice.

A novice meditator should meditate in a quiet place. Anywhere is fine. The best environment for meditation is "a place where I can be quiet and

かで「自分が今私自身のために静かになれる処」それが瞑想の環境です。

　ある人は、専用の瞑想ルームを自宅に造りました。自宅の庭先の２畳ほどの絨毯敷きの個室です。そこは照明もコントロールでき、音楽も聴けるような装置も配置して、本格的な瞑想環境を演出しています。またマンションの一室を瞑想ルームにしている方もいます。ここまでくればホンモノでしょうが、一般の方にとって、瞑想ルームなどは願ってもなかなか手に入りません。

　でも大丈夫です。瞑想は、専用の部屋がなくてもいろんな工夫次第でなんとでもなります。大家族で暮らしていても静かな時間は、あなた次第で作れるのです。自宅あるいは公園、あるいは職場の空き部屋、どこでもいいので自分なりにひとりになれて、その空間が誰にも邪魔されず、少しの時間を確保できる場所であればOKです。

　ただし、坐るために身体のバランスなどを考えると、比較的水平が確保されているとこをお奨めします。瞑想する場所が傾いていては、気持ちや心も定まりません。野外で瞑想するときも、なるべく平坦な場所を選んで行うのが効果的です。ヨーガの行法の作法として「安定した、快適な場所で瞑想をすべき」という定めがあります（ヨーガスートラ）。

　編者は仏教の修行時代には山野に寝起きしたこともあります。また四国巡礼のお遍路をして歩いたときは、海辺の海岸や草原などを選びました。また山の中では、見晴らしが利くところや山の頂上、谷川のほとりで悠々と流れる水の音を聞きながら深い瞑想に入った事もあります。スリランカで初期仏教瞑想をトレーニングしたときは、僧院内だけでなく、ヤシの樹の下や、広葉樹の木々の木陰で瞑想しました。自然の空気を感じながらの瞑想は格別なものがあります。

　室内であれ、板敷きでも絨毯でもなんでもかまいません。ただし、床の色は好みもありますが、暖色を用いると安らげる傾向にあります。これもカラーセラピー的な視点から論じ始めると、難しくなりますが、要は自分にとって落ち着ける環境づくりを心がけていただければいいのです。

　「今わたしが座っている場所は、とても安心できるところなのだ」と最初に自分に言い聞かせられるところであれば、それでいいのです。

feel at peace in the present moment" in your everyday life.

I know a person who built a meditation room in a garden next to his house, a small carpeted room (about 70 square feet) including lighting and audio systems to create a quality meditative ambience. Another person converted a full room in his apartment into a meditation room. Not everyone, however, can have a dedicated meditation room. In fact, it is okay not to have one. Even if you live with a large family, you can always find somewhere for quiet time for yourself. You can practice meditation wherever you can be alone and not disturbed by anyone for a while. For example, you could use a corner in your house, a park, an unused room in your workplace, etc.

Nevertheless, it is recommended that you sit on a flat surface for meditation. If the surface is inclined, your body and mind will not feel at ease, especially as time progresses. Traditional rules for the practice of Yoga recommends that you should meditate in a stable and comfortable place.

I slept and rose in nature during my training years. When I travelled on the Shikoku Pilgrimage route, I meditated deeply on the beach, a grassy plain, mountaintops and open spaces with commanding views, and on riverbanks with the sound of flowing water. When I practiced Early Buddhist styles of Meditation in Sri Lanka, I meditated not only in monasteries, but in the shade of trees. It was special to meditate in the fresh air.

It does not matter whether you meditate outdoors or indoors, on a wooden floor or carpet. Generally speaking, you can stay calmer on a floor with warm colors, though each person may have their own preferences. The bottom line is that you create an environment that is relaxing for you. It is perfectly fine, so long as you can say, "Right now I am sitting in a very comfortable and safe place."

●用便は済ませておくに限る

　場所が決まったら、次にはお手洗いを事前に済ませておくことが肝心です。膀胱が満ちていては三昧に入りにくいので、身体の反応として用便を済ませておいてください。瞑想の途中で心が安定し、三昧が深まってきたときに、尿意もよおすようでは、集中が半減してしまいます。

　大便はもちろんですが、小便についてはその人の日ごろのパターンがあるでしょうから、時間に配慮して事前の用便を心がけてください。瞑想に関する手引書などでは、この用便についてあまり触れられていませんが、実は専門的な瞑想修行をしていくためには、おろそかにはできないことです。私の経験ですが、仏教（密教）の特別修行を行うときは、1回の堂籠もりが長時間にわたることもあって、調整を誤ると大変苦労をします。それはお堂に入るときには、1回ごとに沐浴（水をかぶる）をするために、用便した場合も再度沐浴して身を清めてからでないと堂内に入れないからです。

　夏ならまだしも、高野山時代の修行では真冬の氷点下で行います。1日2食（精進の粗食）での修行で1回の用便と沐浴に費やす時間と体力消耗を考えると、なるべく堂内にはいったら動かないほうがいいのです。

　あなたに専門的な修行をしなさいといっているのではありません。もし在家（出家しないで一般家庭で生活すること）のままであっても、将来において瞑想を生活に取り入れ、ある程度専門的な瞑想ライフを生きようとするならば、はじめから瞑想前の用便の習慣はつけておいたほうがいいということです。

　つまり瞑想とは、不安材料を極力少なくして、自分のための「安心の時間と空間づくりを生活習慣としてマスターすること」なのです。このことはいろんなライフスタイルに応用されますので、最初は意識して心がけるようにしてください。

●服装はリラックスできるものが一番

　服装に決まったものはありません。基本的にはあなたが選ぶなら、どのよ

· Go to the bathroom

After you pick a place for meditation, you should go to the bathroom. To enter a state of concentration called Samadhi, one should take care of the biological needs of bladder and bowel, before starting to meditate, preventing needing to interrupt your meditation session and unnecessary distractions, allowing you to maintain your concentration during the session.

Although this point is rarely mentioned in meditation textbooks, it's importance for specialized meditation practice and should not be underestimated! Meditation means creating a peaceful time and place for yourself as part of your daily routines, and this includes attending to bodily functions that might end up distracting you.

• Wearing loose and comfortable clothing

There is no rule about clothing for meditation. You can choose whatever you prefer. One thing to keep in mind, though, is to wear loose-fitting (comfortable) clothes. Pants without a tight belt are good. One aim of meditation is to "let your mind be flexible and release worldly attachments." If your body feels constrained, so will your mind. This is why I do not recommend tight clothes or underwear that makes sitting difficult. Casual clothes like T-shirts are perfectly fine. What is important is that you can breathe easily, and that your shoulders and legs do not feel constrained.

In a way, meditation creates an "extraordinary time" to elevate one's mind and spirit. Therefore, it is very effective to meditate by giving special significance to this extraordinary time. You might motivate yourself by changing into your own chosen meditation outfit and telling yourself that "meditation begins now." I, for one, feel best in Samue (作務衣), the comfortable and loose working clothes traditionally for Japanese Buddhist priests.

うな格好で瞑想をしようと、それは自由です。服装で注意すべき点は、体を
いたずらに締め付けないようにするということです。ベルトなどもなるべく
しなくてすむようなズボンやスラックスがいいでしょう。もともと「こころ
に柔軟性をもち、いろいろな執着心を手放す」ことが瞑想の目的でもあるの
で、体の窮屈は心の窮屈につながるので、坐りづらい服装はあまりお奨めで
きません。下着もあまり締め付けないようなものがいいですね。現代はいろ
んな服装がありますから、こだわらずラフな服装でいいのです。Tシャツで
かまいません。大切なことは呼吸が十分に確保されて、肩にも脚にも窮屈さ
を感じないラフな格好が一番なのです。

　最近は瞑想時に作務衣を着て、日常とは違う気持ちで瞑想を楽しむ人が増
えています。これは大変結構なことだと思います。ある意味で、瞑想は日常
ではない時間、つまり「非日常」の時間を確保して、自分のために心やスピ
リチュアリティを高めることですから、非日常の時空に特別な意味や意義を
もたせて瞑想することはとても有用なことです。

　自分なりの瞑想コスチュームに着替えて、「これから瞑想だ」と自分に言
い聞かせて始めるのも動機づけとしていいかもしれません。

　出家者は、法衣のままで瞑想する訓練をしてきましたので、やはり作務衣
が一番楽なのです。

２）瞑想の開始

・６つの座法、ただしどれでもいい

　瞑想の姿勢は基本的には静座（背筋を伸ばして静かに座ること）です。坐っ
て背筋が伸びる状態を保てれば瞑想に入れます。瞑想前に軽い柔軟体操をし
ておくことも、心身のバランスをとる意味ではとても大切なことです。

　しかし、病気などや障害があってどうしても坐っていられない方は、仰臥
位として寝そべったままで瞑想もできます。ただ人は横になって、深い呼吸
をするとリラックスしてそのまま、睡眠に入ってしまうことがありますので、
瞑想前には十分に睡眠をとっておくことが肝要です。

2) Beginning meditation

• Sitting

Basically, you meditate by sitting calmly with your back straight. It is often useful to do some light movements or stretches to balance your body and mind just before sitting. Those who cannot sit on the floor due to physical limitations may meditate lying on their back. However, deep breathing and relaxation when lying on the floor tend to induce sleep. It is therefore important to get enough sleep before meditation.

Buddhist priests in Japan used to strictly instruct newcomers on how to sit in meditation halls, but some of them have become lenient because lifestyles and habits changed. Nowadays, more people meditate in a comfortable position with the help of chairs or sofas. Nonetheless, some denominations still instruct strictly. If you learn from teachers from those denominations, you should follow your teacher's instructions. Note that various sitting styles historically existed, and irrespective of style, the substance is what is more important.

There are six basic ways of sitting for meditation, from which you can choose whichever one feels more comfortable.

① Kekkafuza 結跏趺坐 (Lotus position蓮華座): Cross-legged sitting, with each foot positioned on top of the opposite leg's thigh, as you might see in many traditional pictures of meditation. (see fig.2,3)

② Hankaza 半跏坐 (Half-lotus position半蓮華座): Sitting with one foot placed on the opposite thigh. (see fig.4)

③ Yamatoza 大和坐: Sitting by opening your knees outwardly slightly off the ground, while the hands each grasp a knee. It is among the most popular sitting styles in Japan. (see fig.5)

④ Sitting on a chair with your back straight. It is easy for modern

Section 2. Meditation●33

最近は、日本人でも正座をする習慣がないために、畳や床にちゃんと坐れない人が多くなりました。昔は僧堂で座法については厳しく指導しましたが、近年は生活習慣の違いから、あまりやかましくいわないところもあります。むしろ瞑想そのものが大事ですから、その人なりに工夫して椅子やソファーを利用した楽な姿勢の瞑想愛好者が増えているようです

　仏教の宗派によっては、いまも厳格に姿勢を指導しているところもありますから、その瞑想指導者の指示に従うようにしてください　本来の瞑想は、中味が肝心です。スタイルについては、歴史的にもさまざまな教えがあることを理解してください。

　整理しますと座法には、次の6通りがあります。
①結跏趺坐（蓮華座）：両足を互い大腿部の上部に乗せて組むこと
②半跏坐（半蓮華座）：片方の足を、一方の大腿部の上部に乗せて組むこと
③大和坐：アグラをかくが足を組まない（一番多い姿勢）
④イスに坐って静座を保つ（現代人にはやりやすい）
⑤正座をする
⑥仰臥位になって、姿勢を穏やかに保つ

　はじめに2、3回大きく手を上部に挙げて背伸びをするといいでしょう。はじめから背筋が曲がって、不自然な格好で瞑想しても、長い時間を保つ事ができませんし、瞑想へのモチベーションが長続きしません。

　どのような座法でもかまいませんが、肝心なのは、導入時に「背筋を伸ばして、呼吸と意識の流れをしっかり確認する」ことです。ゆっくりと口から吐いて、それからゆっくりと鼻から吸ってください。

　最初はなるべく基本に添って行うことを心がけてください。実はそれが早く上達し、瞑想が自分のものになる秘訣でもあります。座具も座布団だけでなく、薄いクッションを重ねたり、低反発座具などを利用したりして、自分の体型に適合するモノを用意することが大事です。

瞑想のための坐法　How to sit for Meditation

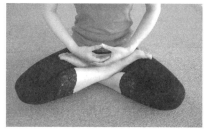

図2(fig.2)　結跏趺坐①（Kekkafuza ①）

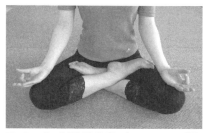

図3(fig.3)　結跏趺坐②（Kekkafuza ②）

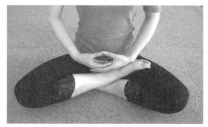

図4(fig.4)　半跏坐（Half-seated）

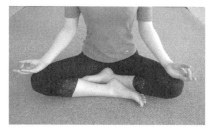

図5(fig.5)　大和座（Yamatoza）

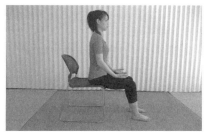

図6(fig.6)　椅子（Chair seat）

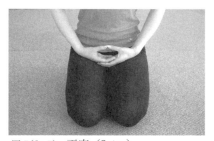

図7(fig.7)　正座（Seiza）

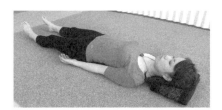

図8(fig.8)　仰臥位（Supine position）

• 手の位置

さらに、瞑想中の手の位置については、仏像のようにさまざまな形が示されています。

一番ポピュラーな手印は、法界定印という形です。手の甲を下にして左手の上に右手をのせます。そして左右の親指を中心で合わせます。（図 2,4,7）これは胎蔵界の大日如来の印でもあります。最初に丹田となる位置、ちょうどお臍のあたりに置いて、深い呼吸とともに気を充実させます。その後に肩や腕の力を抜くように、息を吐くと同時に、組んでいる手を下に落ちるまで、ストンと納めます。

無理のない自然な形を習得してください。

手を膝頭で左右に広げた印もあります。現代人は、ヨーガを学ぶ講座でこの印を知ることも多いかと思います。この広げるやり方にもそのまま手の平を上に向けて、そのまま指を自然に伸ばして広げる方法もあれば、親指と人差し指でリングをつくり、他の指は伸ばします。その手の甲を膝頭につけて伸ばすのも多く見られるスタイルです。（図 3,5,6）

指でつくったリングは、手の平で受け止めた大自然のエネルギーを、指のところで増幅して体内に取り込むコイルのはたらきもします。そういうイメージで瞑想をすることに意味があります。

たとえば、「わたしは今、大自然のエネルギーを全身で受けてパワーアップしている」というイメージ効果です。

正座をしたままの瞑想では手の位置は、おのずと膝の上に置くことになります。無理のない自然な形を習得してください。

• 3種の目線

仏像の表情には、眼を開けているのか閉じているのかわからないようなものもあります。瞑想の時の目線にも、手印と同じようにそれぞれに意味があります。結論から言うと、実は瞑想の目線には、

①半眼にして、1、2メートル先の床を見続ける半眼瞑想
②眼を閉じたままでいる閉眼瞑想

people. (see fig.6)

⑤ Seiza 正座: Sitting on your calves and feet, bent at the knees beneath you. (see fig.7)

⑥ Supine position: Lying calmly on your back. (see fig.8)

You may stretch your body, raising both your hands several times before you meditate. With poor posture, your motivation for continuing the meditation will decrease, and the session will not last long. You may choose any posture. What is important is to straighten your spine and be aware of your breath and stream of consciousness in starting meditation.

Beginners should follow the aforementioned basic postures, which are key to making progress and mastering meditation. In addition to a sitting mat, it may be helpful to have additional props that work for your body, such as a thick floor cushion, a double layered thin cushion or a low rebounding cushion.

• **Hand position**

There are various hand positions during meditation as you might see in various statues of Buddha. The most popular Buddhist hand position is called Hokaijo-in (法界定印). You turn up your palms, place your right hand on your left, and joint the tips of both thumbs. You then place your hands in front of the "Tanden (丹田)," the center of your abdomen, and breathe deeply and concentrate your attention on consciousness. (see fig.2,4,7) Later you relax your shoulders and arms and drop your hands naturally to your legs when breathing out.

In another posture, you place your open hands on your knees. Many of you may come across this hand position in yoga classes. To create this hand position, you may extend your arms with your palms up and your fingers slightly and naturally curved as your hands rest upon your knees. Alternatively, you may create a circle with your thumb and forefinger

③眼を開けたままで何かに集中する開眼瞑想、の３種類があります。

　半眼瞑想とは、床面を見つめるのではなく、注意を自己の心に集中するために、漠然と見つめるだけです。さらにこの方法は、眼を閉じて行うのに比べて、瞑想中に睡眠に入ってしまうのを防ぐ意味もあります。

　閉眼瞑想は、半眼よりもっと自己の内面を観察し洞察するときに、集中しやすい状況をつくるのに役立ちます。眼を閉じても、意識としては瞼の裏側を見ている感覚です。こうすることによって、暗闇の中でもしっかり心眼を開き、内面的な意識の有り様を見つめることに有効です。ただ瞑想中に知らず知らずに眠ってしまうことがあるので、要注意です。

　開眼瞑想は、しっかり肉体的視覚を発揮して、対象となる「もの」を見つづけるという瞑想です。この対象となるものとは「光明、仏像、マンダラ、梵字、表象文字、絵画、植物、自然界」などです。これは特にイメージ瞑想に有効で、自分の目標や目的とする何かを確立するとき、あるいはそれを自分の内面に取り入れたいときに活用します。洞察瞑想というよりは希望する自己のセルフイメージを高める方法として大変有効です。

　飛騨千光寺の瞑想道場においては病気の人が心身の恢復を願って、慢性疾患の方やがんの療養中の方が心身の恢復をイメージして瞑想したり、うつ病の方が自己のセルフイメージを高めたりするときに、光の本尊を視て瞑想しています。私は、それによって何人もの方の症状が軽減するのを見てきました。

　目線はその時の瞑想の目的で異なってくるということを、覚えておいてください。

・**自律神経に影響する呼吸法**

　呼吸そのものは本来自然なものですから、規則などはないといってもいいでしょう。人間に限らず生き物は、生きていくためには呼吸をしなくてはなりません。仕方など教わらなくても、誰もが自然に呼吸をしています。ですから、瞑想においても、基本的には自然な呼吸そのものでいいのです。

　しかし、ここで敢えて瞑想のための呼吸法を学べば、瞑想が、より意義深いものであり、また自分自身の新たな優れた自己管理のツール（道具）であ

and other fingers slightly curved, resting the backs of your hands on your knees. (see fig.3,5,6) It is said that making a circle with your thumb and forefinger creates a coil, amplifying the natural energy that you receive through your palms. Having this image in mind during meditation is meaningful. For example, it may be helpful to imagine, "I am taking in the energy of nature through my whole body, and I am empowered."

When meditating in Seiza (正座), you naturally place your hands on your lap.

• **Three States of eyes**

You sometimes cannot tell whether the eyes of Buddhist statues are open or not. There are three positions for the eyes during meditation: open, half-closed, and closed. Different positions have different intentions, just like different hand positions do.

① Half-closed: You vaguely see the floor a few meters ahead. You do not focus on the floor but on your mind or heart. This position also helps you stay awake during meditation.

② Closed: This position better helps increase your focus when focusing and penetrating internally, compared with half-closed eyes. It is as if you were looking at the back of your eyelids. This enables you to keep your mind's eye open in the dark and observe the state of your inner consciousness. However, you have to be careful not to fall asleep during meditation.

③ Open: You meditate by continuously looking at an object with your own eyes. This object is, for example, radiance, a statue of Buddha or another statue with sacred meaning to you, Mandala, ideogram, drawing, a plant or nature, and so on. This position of the eyes is especially effective during "image meditation" to define your goal or purpose and incorporate it into your mind. This meditation and eye position works to elevate your own self-image rather than reflecting on your present self. In the Hida-Senkōji meditation hall, those who have chronic diseases or

ることを発見できます。それはこれまで先人がいろいろな呼吸法を通じて、教えてきたことです。ここでは誰でも実践しやすいものを、私が選んでお伝えしたいと思います。

　ヨーガや仏教でも初心者に対する呼吸法があります。編者は、これまで20年に渡っていろいろな場で瞑想セッションを実施した経験から、ここではできるだけシンプルで効果的なものをお伝えします（図9）。

①まず座法や目線が定まったら、息を口から大きく吐きます。吐き方は口先を前に出して細く長く、遠くに息を飛ばす感覚で吐いてください。最初は自分の体内にはもう息は無いと思えるほど、しっかり最後まで吐ききってください。

②次に、吐ききった反動で、鼻からすうっと息を吸ってください。これは吐くほど長くなくてもいいので、気持ちよく勢いよく体内に入ってくる呼吸を感じてください。

③再び、身体に新鮮な空気が入ってきたと意識して、吸い込んだ空気を大切に①の要領でゆっくり吐いてください。

④この「吐く息」「吸う息」そのものに集中して、7回以上繰り返してください。1回ごとに「ひと～つ、ふた～つ、……」などと呼吸回数をいいながら続けることもいいでしょう。

　なぜ7回なのかというと、はっきりした論拠ではないのですが、「7」という数字に隠された不思議なパワーがあるのです。仏教の真言念誦（マントラ）なども普段は7回唱えることを習慣としてきています。これもまたどうしてかという根拠は明確ではありませんが、どうやらこれくらい行うと、脳波が変化するようです。ちなみに息を吐くときは副交感神経を、吸うときは交感神経を優位に活動させるといわれています。

⑤元来は、この呼吸回数を限定されたのではありません。あなた自身が「こころが落ち着くまで」適宜にやってください。人間はそのときの身体状態や気持ちがいつも同じではありません。瞑想に入る手前の出来事や、さまざまな状況を引きずりながら瞑想に入ることも少なくないでしょう。そのために心

cancer meditate by imagining themselves becoming healthy again, and those who suffer from depression meditate by imagining a central image of radiant Light to enhance their self-image. I have observed many people whose symptoms were relieved by radiance meditation, just one of the many forms of image meditation.

• **How breathing affects the autonomic nervous system**

People breathe naturally since birth without learning how to do so. All living beings, including humans, need to breathe to live. So, during meditation, you can breathe normally. However, if you learn a method of breathing for meditation, you will find meditation more meaningful and turn it into a superior self-management tool. This is what our predecessors have been teaching through various methods of breathing.

Yoga and Buddhism both teach various methods of breathing for beginners. Below, I present the simplest and most effective ways of breathing based on my experience of meditation sessions in various situations during the past twenty years.

① At first, sitting with your back straight, you decide on your posture and eye position. Once settled into position, breathe out deeply through your mouth. By puckering your lips, breathe out as if you were blowing off the air little by little into the long distance. You should breathe out completely as if your lungs had no more air.

② Next, you breathe in from your nose. This inbreath does not have to be as long as your outbreath. Feel the breath comfortably and energetically coming into your body.

③ Being aware of the fresh air coming into your body, breathe out again as you did in ①.

④ You repeat this style of breathing in and out seven times or more. If it

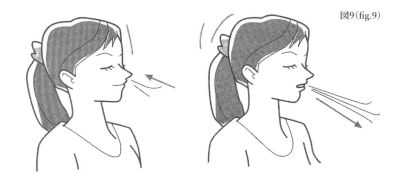

図9(fig.9)

を平安に保つための呼吸法は、そのときによって異なってあたりまえです。

　しかし、ここで瞑想を自分のものにするためのアプローチとして、毎回の導入呼吸時に「私は○回、深い呼吸をすると、心がリセットされて、平安が訪れる」と今を感じながら繰り返しやっていると、いつしかその回数の呼吸法でいつでも心の安らぎを獲得することができるようになります。

⑥深い呼吸法が一段落したら、普通の呼吸に戻します。普段と変わりないリズムの呼吸に戻りますが、少しゆったりとした感覚になって、もはや深い呼吸をする前と今とでは、呼吸の流れも変わっていることに気づきます。

　このあとの呼吸は鼻だけの呼吸で瞑想に入っていきます。つまり鼻から吸って口から吐く、やがて鼻から吸って鼻から吐くという繰り返しです。

3）内面への気づき

・雑念の処理

　「瞑想中の雑念をどうすればよいですか」とは、よく聞かれる質問です。瞑想の初心者で、次々に浮かんでくる雑念に悩まされる人は多いのでしょう。私たち人間は「生(なま)もの」ですから、心身ともに常に運動しており、たとえ身体は動いていなくても、細胞は働き続け、意識も同じように動いています。瞑想中だからといって、すべての動きを完全にストップさせるのは容易なことではありません。しかし、心配はご無用です。訓練で少しずつ調整できる

helps, you can count, "one, two⋯" at every breath. The reason of seven times is unclear, but it is said that the number "seven" has secret and mysterious power. The Shingon nenju mantra (真言念誦) in Buddhism is also conventionally repeated seven times. Chanting seven times may help to make brain waves change. According to some studies, breathing out activates the parasympathetic nervous system and breathing in activates the sympathetic nervous system.

⑤ The number of times you should breathe is not fixed. You may breathe as many times as you need until your mind becomes calm. Physical conditions and mood do not remain constant. You sometimes start meditation by thinking about what happened beforehand or ruminating on other things. It is therefore natural that the method of breathing that can relax your mind varies depending on the circumstances. However, I propose that you tell yourself "I reset my mind and feel calm after I breathe deeply seven times (or the number that suits you)" every time you begin to meditate. You can eventually manage to calm your mind whenever you breathe to the number.

⑥ After you feel settled with deep breathing, you start breathing normally. Even though you breathe with a normal rhythm, you feel more relaxed, and you can also sense that the flow of your breath has changed because of deep breathing. Subsequently, you breathe in and out repeatedly only through your nose. In short, you start by breathing in through your nose and breathing out through your mouth, and then you proceed to breathing in and out only through your nose.

3) Awareness of the inner mind

- **Managing Distracting Thoughts (Zatsunen 雑念)**

I am often asked by beginners, "How do I manage distracting thoughts in

ようになります。

　瞑想入門時に浮かんでくる雑念は、「私には瞑想は向いていないかも……」「瞑想しても集中できないのは私がいけないのかしら」など、多くが不安感からきています。しかし、その判断は早計です。たくさんの雑念に追いかけられるあなたこそ、瞑想が必要な人であり、やがて瞑想の達人になれる資質があるのです。

　雑念は、意識の底から浮かんでくる水泡のようなもので、放っておくと自然に消えていきますから、無理に追い出そうとしたり、無視したりする必要はありません。瞑想中は、自然に浮かんでは消える雑念を、そのまま判断せずに観察しているだけでよいのです。

　また、瞑想中は吐く息と吸う息だけに意識を集中してください。たとえば、「足が痛いな」という雑念が出たら、「呼吸に戻る、呼吸に戻る、呼吸に戻る」と３回ほど自分に言い聞かせることによって呼吸に集中し、雑念から離れます。雑念から集中に戻る訓練を何度も繰り返すことによって、そのうちに雑念に惑わされなくなります。このように呼吸に集中する瞑想を、初期仏教における「シャマタ（止観）瞑想」といいます。

　それでもなかなか消えないしつこい雑念は、「今後私が瞑想によって洞察し、解決する課題かもしれないな」というくらいに留めておき、後でそのことを記録しておきましょう。

　心象風景はその人の深い意識と関係しますが、あるがままにゆったりと受け止めて瞑想を続け、何度も呼吸に戻る訓練を行うことが雑念の対応に有用です。

• 想念の観察

　瞑想のような静かな環境では、雑念と同様に、「普段、自分が気にしていること」が表面意識に現れてくることがあります。これを「想念」といい、ときには想念で頭が一杯になってしまうこともあります。初心者の瞑想では、その想念を「ありのままに観察する」ことを繰り返し実践します。

　要はそのときに浮かんでくる意識をそのまま観察して、「あぁ、今私の中にある思いは、こんなことを感じているのだな」と、自分を冷静に見ている

my mind." Many beginners suffer from one distracting thought after another. Because we are human beings, our bodies and minds are always active. Even when our bodies are not moving, cells and consciousness are working. It is therefore difficult to stop all activities, even during meditation. However, you can begin to manage your thoughts gradually through practice.

At an early stage of meditation practice, your distracting thoughts often come from your anxious feelings like "I'm not very good at meditation..." and "I might be meditating wrong, because I can't concentrate." These judgments are premature. Precisely because you suffer from distracting thoughts, you need meditation—and you have the talent to eventually becoming a meditation expert.

Distracting thoughts are like bubbles of water coming up from the depth of consciousness. If you leave them as they are, they naturally disappear. So, it is unnecessary to try hard to force them out or ignore them. You simply observe the thoughts appearing and disappearing non-judgmentally.

During meditation, you should focus only on your outbreath and inbreath. If the thought of pain in a foot occurs to you, tell yourself, "Come back to the breath, come back to the breath, come back to the breath" three times. Then you will leave the distracting thought and focus on your breath again. This practice of leaving distracting thoughts and focusing on your breath is called Shamata (calm abiding and clear observation) meditation in Early Buddhism. With practice, you will suffer less from distracting thoughts. When distracting thoughts persist, you simply note, "these thoughts may be the issues that I need to penetrate through meditation and resolve in the future." As mental scenery is linked with deep consciousness, you may accept the thoughts as they are and keep meditating by repeating the practice of returning to your breath as an effective response to distracting thoughts.

図10(fig.10)　仏教の深層意識・唯識から密教まで
Composition of human mind by Buddism

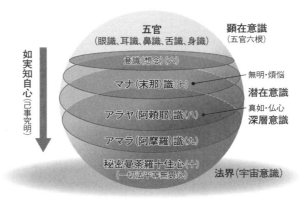

　もう1人の自分を意識化します。そしてすぐに結論を出すことはせず、その想念を注視し、観察し続ける訓練をするのです。
　そのうち、「この思いについては、しばらく様子をみよう」というように、自分なりに思いを受容しながら、次の課題を見つめられるようになります。次々と出てくる想念について、自分にとって今すぐ取り組むべきものなのか、後でもよいのか、ゆっくり観察しましょう。これによって、抱えている課題や難題の交通整理をすることができます。
　雑念も想念も、決して悪いものではありません。仏教心理学の唯識学ではこれらを「マナ（末那）識」といいます。ここには、自分というものを知っていくうえで、とても重要な情報が集まっている、まさに「スピリチュアリティの種」なのです。生きるうえで生ずる悩み、煩悩や雑念は、悟りを目指す種であり、煩悩があるからこそ、悟りを目指す活動があります。このような営みを仏教では「煩悩即菩提」といいます。
　「みつめる瞑想」の重要なプログラムである観察・洞察瞑想は、内面から出てくる事柄から自己を知るために、最初は、自分と他人との間にある境界について、思いを巡らせて観察することが重要になります。
　たとえば、「私がこの世に生まれたとき、両親はどこにいて、どんな生活

- **Observation of Sōnen 想念 (everyday worry)**

Besides Zatsunen 雑念 (distracting thought), Sōnen (everyday worry) often arise at the surface of your consciousness when meditating in quiet environments. These everyday worries or concerns may sometimes preoccupy your mind. Beginners repeatedly observe the worry "as it is" during meditation. The key is that you consider yourself as a clinical observer of your own suffering from everyday worries. You as an observer become aware that "This is how my everyday worries feel like now." Instead of rushing to draw a conclusion, you keep observing the worry. Gradually, you can begin to accept the worry, leave it as it is for a while, and proceed to another task in your life. When one worry arises after another, you need to observe patiently which worry you should take care of now and which you can defer to a later time. This allows you to sort out your problems and challenges.

Zatsunen 雑念 and Sōnen 想念 are not always bad. Those are also known as Manashiki 末那識 (Ego-consciousness) in Yuishiki 唯識 (consciousness-only) Buddhist psychology and are regarded to be "Seeds of spirituality" that contain important information about who you really are. Worries, worldly desires, and distracting thoughts in life can be the seeds of aspiration toward spiritual enlightenment: precisely because of these worldly desires, people can find inspiration for and aspire to enlightenment. This process is called "Bonnō soku bodai 煩悩即菩提 (worldly desire leads immediately to enlightenment)" in Buddhism.

Observing Meditation requires you to consider and observe boundaries between you and others, so that you can know yourself from the issues arising in your inner mind. For example, you look back on and observe your relationship and proximity with people to whom you have become connected. That is, you carefully remember, "When I was born, where did my parents live, how did they make a living?", "Where was my brother or sister?", "How did I grow up in the family?", and so on. This practice makes

をしていたのか。きょうだいはどこにいたのか。私はその中でどんなふうに育ったのか」というように、これまでご縁のあった人との関係性や距離感を振り返って観察します。すると、自分が周りの人々との間にどんな境界をつくっているのか、そのパターンに気づきます。瞑想を通じて、まずはこのような訓練を行ってみることで、内面を洞察する瞑想の入り口が見えてきます。

・安らぎを感じる

瞑想は、慣れないうちは苦しいだけで終わってしまうこともあります。日常の苦しいことやネガティブな事柄ばかりが浮かんでくると、「瞑想なんて、もうイヤ！」と投げ出したくなるかもしれません。それでも瞑想を続けていると、その人なりに安定した境地に達して、ふっと、何ともいえない「安らぎ」「平安」が訪れることがあります。これは、「脳内麻薬」と呼ばれるβエンドルフィンや「幸せホルモン」と呼ばれるセロトニンという神経伝達物質のはたらきでもあり、実は大変重要なメッセージなのです。

瞑想の目標は、「己事究明」（自己とは何者か）という自分探しから始まって、やがて「たかめる瞑想」「ゆだねる瞑想」で大いなる意識との融合に至ることです。この意識状態をトランスパーソナル心理学では「拡張意識」と呼び、仏教では「三昧」「悟り」「覚醒」などと表現しています。[4]

そして、最終目標は「自我」にとらわれる執着から離れることです。達成するのは容易ではありませんが、瞑想中に訪れる安らぎや平安は、自己の執着を手放した後に訪れる意識状態ですから、この最終目標に着実に近づいている証といえるでしょう。

スポーツでもお稽古ごとでも、最初からうまくできる人はいません。ぎこちなくとも諦めずに同じことを続けていると、最初の不自然さがいつの間にか自分の動作に同化して、自然な立ち居振る舞いに変化していることに気づきます。

瞑想も同じです。当初はさまざまな意識の不安定さを自覚して、自己嫌悪に陥り、投げやりになることもありますが、そういうプロセスを通して、やがて瞑想の達人になれるのです。瞑想の安らぎ感を体得することは、あなた自身の魂の成長につながります。

you notice your patterns regarding how you create boundaries between yourself and others. You will thus arrive at the entrance to Observing Meditation by penetrating into the inner depths of your mind.

- **Attaining peace of mind**

Beginners sometimes struggle to meditate because only hardships and negative issues arise in their minds. Many people then feel like giving up on meditation. Nevertheless, those who keep practicing meditation can reach a stable state and unexpectedly attain peace and calm. This likely happens due to the working of neurotransmitters like beta-endorphin, dubbed "intracerebral narcotics," and serotonin "happiness hormones." Beginning with "Kojikyūmei 己事究明 (a journey of self-discovery)," a meditator can then aim to become one with "Something Greater" through "Energizing Meditation" and "Unifying Meditation". Such a state of consciousness is called "expanded consciousness" in transpersonal psychology and "Samādhi (a state of intense concentration achieved through meditation)" in Buddhist traditions.[4] An ultimate goal is to let go of worldly attachments to the ego, a goal not easily attained. However, if you feel peaceful and calm during meditation, you are approaching the final goal because those feelings are the states of consciousness that arise from letting go of the ego.

No one succeeds in the first attempts in any sports or arts. If you continue to practice without giving up, initial awkwardness, discomfort, or uncertainty will be assimilated into natural and smooth movements. Meditation is the same. At first, you become conscious of your mental instability and sometimes become self-critical and desperate. However, many people become experts at meditation through such experiences. Learning how to attain peace of mind by facing those parts of oneself leads to your mental and personal growth.

第3章

4つの瞑想メソッド（実習に向けての理解）

1）ゆるめる瞑想法（緩和、集中型瞑想法）

　一言でいうと意識を「緩和し、集中する」瞑想法です。ゆるめる瞑想は、緩和する瞑想と集中する瞑想からなります。

　緩和とは「心身をゆるめること」で、ゆるんだ状態によって、ニュートラルな意識（中立的な感覚）を取り戻すと、徐々に一点に集中できるようになります。それには、まず身体を徹底してゆるめることを行います。深い呼吸の連続で弛緩状態を維持して、ある程度の休息や睡眠ができたと感じたら、起き上がって座法によるゆるめる瞑想を継続することができます。

　ゆるめる瞑想の大事なことは、まずリラックスして呼吸ができる、ということと静かな気持ちを継続できることです。今の自分の思いや感情を否定しないように、そのまま受け入れることです。

　この2点を、自分がいつでもどこででもできるようになると、心を落ち着けたいと思ったときに実行できます。瞑想の初めは難しいことではなく、ひたすら出入りの呼吸を見続ける訓練をします。

　意図的な呼吸（意識的に息を長く吐くこと）によって身体とのリズムを調和させることができます。息を意識的に吐くことによって、副交感神経の活性化をはかり、脳波をアルファ波が優位な状態にし、脳内の神経伝達物質の分泌を促す効果があることが解明されています。その結果、深い瞑想は身体にさまざまな良い影響をもたらします。

　基本は心身をゆるめると、その後に一点に集中できるようになります。集中する瞑想法は仏教では「シャマタ瞑想」[5]として伝承されています。それは、ひたすら呼吸の出入りに集中する瞑想が中心となります。瞑想の導入部

50●第3章　4つの瞑想メソッド（実習に向けての理解）

Section 3.

Four methods of meditation
(Preparing for meditation practice)

1) "Loosening Meditation" (relief/concentration)

In short, "Loosening Meditation" is a method to relax your body and mind and to concentrate your consciousness. That is, Loosening Meditation consists of Relief meditation and Concentration meditation. When your body and mind are relaxed, consciousness becomes neutral, which makes it easier to concentrate. To create such a condition, you should first fully relax your body and mind. Lying on your back, you maintain relaxation through a series of deep breaths. If you feel rested enough, you can rise up and continue Loosening Meditation while sitting.

The essence of Loosening Meditation is to be able to feel relaxed with peaceful breaths and maintain a sense of calm. You may accept yourself as you are without denying your thoughts and feelings. It is a process, but if you can ultimately manage to be relaxed with peaceful breaths and to keep a calm feeling anytime and anywhere, you can calm your heart whenever necessary. The first part of Loosening Meditation is to only observe breathing in and breathing out. This is not difficult. Breathing out consciously for a long time harmonizes the rhythms of body and mind. According to some studies, a conscious and long outbreath activates the parasympathetic nervous system, makes alpha waves dominant, and stimulates secreting neurotransmitters in the brain. That is, deep meditation has various positive effects on health.

分で心身の弛緩状態を十分に確認すると、のちに「集中」という精神状態が起きてきます。安定した精神状態が出現すると、集中瞑想の状態になるのです。これを三昧(サマーディー)状態と表現することもあります。三昧状態は、初期仏教では9つの段階を教えています。その最終を「無相」といいます。

　呼吸の出入りに注視して、「私は今、息を吐いている」「私は今、息を吸っている」というように、ひたすら呼吸そのものに集中するのです。「足が痛いな」「寒いな」「明日の仕事は……」などと、次々に雑念が起こってきても「呼吸に戻る」「呼吸に戻る」「呼吸に戻る」と、何度も自分に言い聞かせて呼吸の出入りに集中します。これがシャマタ瞑想の訓練なのです。

　編者は、1980年にスリランカのテーラーヴァーダー（上座部仏教）の寺院で約半年の瞑想生活をしました。そのとき、年配の僧侶がこの集中瞑想を理解するコツを教えてくれました。それは「私は今、樹をみている」「私は今、樹の葉をみている」「私は今、ゆっくり歩いている」というように、ひたすら「ありのままの今を感じて、呼吸を継続する」ことだと教えてくれました。

　さらに歩く瞑想は集中力を養う訓練には最適です。まさにマインドフルネスなのです。次の段階は、自分の今感じている心や感情を知ることです。呼吸の出入りを注視して、「私は今、息を吐いている」「私は今、息を吸っている」「いま私は足をあげている」「いま私は足を降ろしている」と、ひたすら足の動きと呼吸そのものに集中します。

　瞑想のはじめは難しいことではなく、ひたすら出入りの呼吸を見続ける訓練をすることなのです。

　日本仏教の本山の1つ高野山では、この集中瞑想を習得するために「阿息観」が実践されています。

　阿息観とは、梵字の阿字を目の前に置いて（図11。図絵がない場合は心でイメージ）しながら、最初に息を吸っておいて、吐く呼吸に「ア〜」、「ア〜」、「ア〜」、「ア〜」、「ア〜」というように声を出すことです。声を出すことで今の呼吸に集中します。吸うときにも阿字を心に観じながら行います。段階的に無声で行うともっと集中瞑想が促進します。ゆるぎない集中瞑想に入ることができるようになると、何も考えないでこの状態を保持することができます。

Concentration meditation has been passed down as "Shamata meditation" [5] in Buddhism. You only focus on breathing in and out in some traditions of Shamata meditation. Fully relaxing your body and mind at the beginning of meditation leads to concentration. Once the mind is stabilized, Concentration meditation begins, which is sometimes described as the state of Samādhi 三昧. According to Early Buddhism, Samādhi has nine stages, the highest of which is called Muso 無相 (free from desires).

During Shamata meditation you can single-mindedly focus on breathing in and out. Even if distracting thoughts, such as "I have leg pain", or "I feel cold", or "Tomorrow I need to work on...", appear one after another, you repeatedly tell yourself, "Focus on breathing in and out", "Focus on breathing in and out", "Focus on breathing in and out." This is the practice of Shamata meditation.

When I practiced meditation for half a year at a Theravada temple in Sri Lanka in 1980, an older priest taught me key points in understanding Shamata meditation: just feel the present moment as it is while continuing to breathe, silently saying to yourself, "I am watching the tree right now", "I am watching the leaf of the tree right now", "I am walking slowly right now", and so on.

Walking meditation is one of the best ways to cultivate concentration. While only focusing on steps and breaths, you tell yourself, "I am breathing in right now", "I am breathing out right now", "I am raising my foot right now", and "I am lowering my foot right now". This is mindfulness and the key in Loosening Meditation.

At Kōyasan, which is the head temple of Esoteric Buddhism in Japan, a method of meditation called "Asokkan 阿息観" is practiced to learn concentration. "Asokkan" means breathing in and breathing out while chanting "Ah", "Ah", "Ah", "Ah" while sitting in front of a scroll of the Sanskrit character "A" and focusing on it. You concentrate on breathing out

Section 3.　Four methods of meditation (Preparing for meditation practice)●53

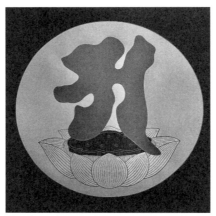

図11(fig.11)　阿字観本尊
"A"character of Bonji (Siddham script)

これも三昧状態です

　ゆるめて集中する瞑想は、最初のうちは5分、10分、15分の瞑想を段階的に繰り返すと、集中瞑想に慣れて、そのうち時間が気にならなくなります。

　慣れてくれば30分、40分の瞑想が自然に行えるようになるのです。最初はぎこちなくとも、続けるということが大切です。

2）みつめる瞑想法（観察、洞察瞑想法）

　みつめる瞑想は、観察瞑想と洞察瞑想からなります。観察瞑想は、あなたを含めたなにかを客観的にあるがままに観察することを意味します。観察瞑想から洞察瞑想への進歩は、初級から中級へと移るようなものです。洞察瞑想は、物事の正しい意味を理解するために、見たり考えたり話したりすることを吟味することを意味します。

　自分の心身に起きている事実を、ありのままに認識するのが観察瞑想です。これはゆるめる瞑想の延長にあります。出入りの呼吸を観察し続けることがその導入になっています。

with vocalization. When you breathe in, you mentally picture the "A-syllable" character. You gradually phase out your voice, deepening concentration meditation in silence. Once concentration meditation is firmly established, you can maintain it effortlessly. This is also a form of Samādhi.

Repeatedly practice Loosening Meditation for five minutes at first. You can gradually increase your meditation time to ten minutes, and then to fifteen minutes. Soon, once you are accustomed to Concentration meditation, you no longer think much about the length of meditation. You become able to meditate for more than thirty to forty minutes naturally. It is important to keep practicing despite any initial awkwardness.

2) "Observing Meditation" (watching/insight)

Observing Meditation consists of Watching meditation and Insight meditation. Watching meditation means to observe things including yourself as they really are. To progress from Watching meditation to Insight meditation is like transitioning from an introductory course to an intermediate one. Insight meditation means to examine the acts of seeing, thinking, and speaking in order to understand the deeper meaning of things.

You can practice Watching meditation by means of recognizing what occurs in your body and mind as it is. Watching meditation is an extension of Loosening Meditation, for it begins with the continuous observation of breathing in and out.

You observe "your position in the family and in society", "complex tasks and challenges", "interpersonal relationships" in your ordinary life, as well as "negative aspects of self-consciousness", "traumatic events", "vulnerabilities" and "pessimisms" in the deepest layer of your mind. You observe them as they are. This is the work through which you carefully

あなたが観察するのは、普段の生活における「家庭や社会での自分の位置」「複雑な仕事や課題」「対人関係」「ネガティブな自意識」や、深層意識に潜む「トラウマ的な出来事」「自分の弱さ」「悲観的感情」などの人生の課題でもあります。それをありのままに観察します。

　さまざまな事実確認を自分の意識や心で丁寧にみていく作業といえるでしょう。このとき「自己の本質的な心理状態を客観的にみることができる位置におく」ということが訓練のポイントとなります。人間は感情的な生き物ですから、第三者として自分をみることが苦手です。どうしても自己防衛が働き、感情移入してしまい、自己を正当化したくなります。

　右手の親指と人差し指で、自分の左手の甲をつまみ上げてみてください。痛いですよね。ここで観察です。「痛みを感じる自分の手の甲」と「痛いという自分の意識」の両方を観察し続けるのです。やがて痛みが徐々に和らいでいくのを感じることができます。

　痛みは脳神経が判断します。しかし痛みの現象を客観的に観察しようとすると、事実を確認した意識が「そんなに命にかかわる大げさな痛みではない」と判断し、あるいは痛みを和らげる神経伝達物質を分泌して痛みが和らいでいきます。このような訓練が、「悩む私」をじっくり観察する基礎をつくってくれます。

　観察瞑想では自我意識をいったん解放して、どこまでも今の自分をありのままに、第三者的に客観的にみていきます。たとえば、問題の所在が自分ではなく相手にあったとしても、その人のせいにするのではなく、そのときの自分の心に起きているさまざまな感情などを、もう1人の自分がしっかり観察するのです。

　これを繰り返すことによって、自己を第三者的にみる習慣ができ、その後の洞察瞑想に入りやすくなります。

　観察瞑想を上手に行うコツは、最初に徹底して「1つの対象を見続ける訓練」をすることです。たとえばりんごを目の前に置いて、ひたすら見続ける訓練をします。りんごの色、形、ツヤなどを細かく観察するのです。うまくできるようになると、ありのままの自分の今の心や過去の心（行動と思念）

examine various facts in your mind and consciousness. The key to this work is to put yourself in the position where you can observe the essence of your mental conditions objectively.

People often have difficulty in seeing themselves objectively because humans are emotional beings and we tend to justify ourselves. One way to observe yourself objectively is to use a little bit of pain. That is, you pinch the back of your hand and observe it. You feel a pain. Then, you keep observing both the back of your hand feeling the pain and your awareness of the pain. Gradually, you can feel the pain is getting relieved. This happens because your cranial nerves judge that the pain is trivial or they secrete neurotransmitters to relieve the pain. Such a training forms the foundation of careful observation of the "worried self."

In Watching meditation, you abandon the ego-consciousness and observe yourself as it is from the third-person perspective. Even when you think another person caused a problem, you do not blame them, but instead carefully observe various feelings that occur in your mind. By repeating this practice, you can acquire the habit of objectively seeing yourself, which makes it easier for you to subsequently enter Insight meditation.

The key to practicing Watching meditation well is to first concentrate on the training of continuing to watch one object. For example, you place an apple in front of you and keep watching it. You only watch the color, shape or glossy surface of the apple in detail. When you become good at this, you can also observe your present and past behaviors and thoughts as they really are.

After you become able to practice Watching meditation, you move to Insight meditation. Insight meditation corresponds to Buddhist teachings known as the Four Noble Truths (Shitai 四諦) and meditations on Right view, Right intension and Right speech, which are all part of the "fourth truth", known as the Eightfold Path (Hasshōdō 八正道). The Insight with

を観察することができるようになります。

観察瞑想がある程度できるようになったら、次は洞察瞑想です。

洞察瞑想は、仏教では「四諦の観察と八正道における正見、正思、正語の瞑想」に該当します。四諦は「生、老、病、死」の命題を、自分の存在性や人生の意味や価値において深い思索をめぐらすことです。たとえば、「何故私は、誰々を両親としてこの世に生まれたのか」、「自分が病気になったり、歳をとったりするのはどんな意味があるか」、「自分の死とはなにか、死ぬまでにやっておきたいことは何か」などと、思惟してみることです。

諦とは「あきらかにみること」であり、物事の実態を正しく理解するために「見ること、思うこと、語ること」を吟味していくことです。物事を正しく純粋に判断できれば、いつでも生死を手放せるのです。瞑想は、観察瞑想で得た「家庭や社会における今の自分の位置」や「厭世感」などの課題について、その出発点まで遡って、原因と結果の有様をゆっくりとみていく作業です。原因究明をしっかりと行う必要があるので、ここでも冷静で客観的な視座が求められます。

怒りや悲しみなどの感情があまりにも強く現れるときは、深い洞察はできません。まだ客観的にみることができない意識状態ということを認識し、その場合は、少し時間をおきクールダウンしてから再度行うといいでしょう。

• みつめる瞑想のヒントとなるワーク

物事を第3者的な視点で観察し、その内面を観ていく洞察を促進するワークがあります。

コンビニエンスストアなどで、容易に手に入るレーズンかナッツを用意します。それを瞑想参加者に、2粒ずつ配ります。最初は普通に1粒を食べます。食べたときの想いを確認します。

次に、1粒を手に取って、形や匂いなどをしっかりと観察します。そして、その果実が「どこの産地で、どんな人に育てられて、どんなふうに成長して、どんな人たちに収穫されたのか、どんなふうに工場に運ばれ、どんなふうに海を渡り、日本の流通に乗ってコンビニまで運ばれ、誰が買って、今目の前

the Four Noble Truths includes observation of Suffering, the Cause of Suffering, the Cessation of Suffering and the Path to the Cessation of Suffering. The first part of "The four noble truths" also asks us to contemplate "The Four Noble Truths – birth, old age, sickness, and death" in light of one's existence and the meaning we give to our life. For example, you ponder "Why was I born in this world to those parents?", "What is the meaning of my becoming ill and old?", "What is the meaning of my death?", "What do I hope to do until I die?" and so on.

"Tai 諦" of Shitai means "clearly seeing," and more specifically, to examine the acts of seeing, thinking and speaking in order to understand the proper meaning of things. You are far more likely to be able to let go of attachments toward life and death if you can properly and genuinely discern things. Insight meditation is the work through which you slowly trace the causes and effects in the issues and challenges like "your position in family and society" or "your pessimism" that you identified during Watching meditation. You have to observe things calmly and objectively because you need to thoroughly investigate the causes.

When you feel strong anger or grief, you cannot practice deep Insight meditation. Then, you need to recognize that you cannot objectively observe things yet, and you may try to meditate again after taking time to cool down.

• **An exercise to help you develop Observing Meditation**

Here is an exercise for improving insight, an act of objectively and deeply observing things:

① Participants of a meditation session receive two raisins.

② First, each participant eats one raisin normally and observes thoughts when eating.

③ Next, each participant picks up another raisin and carefully observes

にあるのか」というように思いを巡らしてから口に入れます。果実の願いや思いのようなものを感じ取って口に入れ、しっかりと味わいます。最後にワークを終えてから、感じたことをお互いに分かち合うこと（シェアリング）によって、それぞれの想いを相互に確認し学ぶことができます。

　一粒の果実を観察し、洞察をめぐらすという一連のプロセスが、この瞑想の学びになるのです。

　この思考法を応用して、自分が生まれたときから成人になるまでの人生のプロセスを洞察します。心理療法やスピリチュアルケア訓練では「生育歴分析」と呼ばれる訓練法です。肝心なのは、あらゆる人生模様に意味づけができて、その人らしく生きられるような「ゆるぎない平安な私のこころ」をつくり出すことです。これは、最終的に自己のスピリチュアリティの成長を促すという意味で、洞察瞑想の大きな目的の1つといえます。

　洞察瞑想は、自分が課題とするものの原因と結果の姿や、将来の方向性を見続けることですから、深く掘り下げる訓練がとても重要です。洞察が進むと、日常の行動の中でも、すぐに洞察的思惟が起こって行動を調整してくれます。

•みつめる瞑想のエクササイズ

　このように観察とは自らの内面世界を客観視することなのです。誰でも、生育歴にはさまざまなエピソードがあります。楽しい思い出もあれば、決して思い出したくないネガティブな記憶もあります。トラウマになるような、つらい思い出もあるかもしれません。さらにそれらの過去の現象を思い出すと、そのときの感情がよみがえり、あるいは付きまとって、苦しい気持ちになります。

　実はここに洞察瞑想の目的があり、目指すべき方向性も示されているのです。苦しい出来事を冷静に見続ける勇気が必要です。

　エクササイズとして、ネガティブな過去とポジティブな過去を1つずつ選んで、観察、洞察瞑想をするという方法があります。

　これは個人でもできるエクササイズですが、グループ（集団）で一緒に瞑

the shape and smell it. They imagine, "Where did the vine grow? Who harvested and dried the grape? How was it processed, distributed and lined up in the convenience store?" and hold it in their mouth and taste it by feeling the raisin's desire and heart.

④ After the exercise, participants share their thoughts and learn from each other.

One can learn to gain clues to Insight meditation even by means of experiencing the process of observing and reflecting on one raisin.

Using the same procedure, you penetrate into your life from your birth to adulthood. This is a training method called "life history analysis" in psychotherapy or training in spiritual care. This practice can help give meaning to your life and cultivate a more stable and peaceful mind. This is an important goal of Insight meditation in the sense of facilitating spiritual growth. In Insight meditation, it is important to practice digging deep into your heart as you must keep penetrating into the causes and effects of your challenges and future direction. Once your insight deepens, you can more easily attain insight in your everyday life to manage your behaviors.

- **Exercise for Observing Meditation**

As described above, observation means taking an objective view of yourself. Everyone has various episodes in his or her life history. Some are happy memories, others are heart-breaking. There might be traumatic and dreadful memories. When recalling them, you may relive the same emotions and feel trapped and distressed by them. Actually, this indicates the purpose of insight meditation and points to the right way to go. You need courage to keep calmly observing hardships.

There is an exercise: you pick a positive past event and a negative past event, and you practice observing and insight meditations with them. You can do this exercise by yourself, but group meditation practice can be more

想会をすると楽しく、学びが大きく効果的に進めることができます。集団で行うことによって、互いの瞑想の内容について、意見交換（シェア）などができて、瞑想の味わいを比較することもできます。

　グループで行う場合は、場所を広くとり、座る間隔を広げるような工夫も大事です。集団瞑想は2、3人の少人数で実施する場合と、10人以上で実施する場合には、空間性や環境に配慮することが大切です。

　最後にメンバー内全体でのシェアによって、さらにお互いの理解が深まります。このときには個人情報にはなるべく触れないで、「この成育歴瞑想でどんな気づきがあったか」を言い合うことが肝心です。それによって、他人がどんな洞察瞑想をしたかを知ることにもなり、瞑想向上の参考になるのです。

　1人で行う場合は、自己の気づきについて、スーパーバイザー（瞑想リーダー）と分かち合うと独善な瞑想にならずに、適切な進展が見られます。

　これらの観察、洞察瞑想を効果的に進めるための方法として、それぞれの出来事をまずテーブルに乗せるということがあります（パソコンのデスクトップに上げるような感覚）。

　「観察瞑想」では、自分を中心に、その場面で関係する人間模様を配置してみます。これはユング心理学の「家族布置（ファミリーコンステレーション）」を参考に、エピソードとなる自分の位置や相手の位置、その距離感や親密性をみることによって、その人との関係性を観察できます。

　「洞察瞑想」では、そのときの自分の具体的な感情や想いを思い出します。次に「関係する人々の想いを相手の立場にたって、思いをめぐらしてみる。そのときに相手の気持ちを感じた自分がどんな気持ちになるか、そこから何に気づくか」というように、洞察するのです。

　こういう自己洞察を0〜5歳、5〜10歳、10〜15歳、15〜20歳、20〜30歳、30〜40歳、40〜50歳、50〜60歳、60歳〜というように年齢的な区切りをもって、父、母、きょうだい、祖父母、親類、友人、先生、会社の同僚などを順番に洞察すると、自己覚知に大きな成果があります。

beneficial to advance your learning effectively and gain deeper knowledge. In a group session, you can exchange and share experiences of meditation with other participants and compare your experience of meditation with others.

In the case of having a group session, it is necessary to have a sufficient and comfortable personal space between sitting participants. Different spaces are necessary for a group of a few participants and that of more than ten. An appropriate space and environment should be prepared corresponding to the numbers of participants in a group session.

【An example meditation session】

① You recall one negative past event for five minutes.

② You penetrate into the negative past event for fifteen minutes.

③ Participants share their experiences with each other.

④ You recall one positive past event for five minutes.

⑤ You penetrate into the positive past event for fifteen minutes.

⑥ Next, a pair of participants share their experiences. Take turns talking for fifteen minutes and listening for fifteen minutes.

⑦ Finally, all participants share their experiences with the larger group.

This final sharing helps deepen mutual understanding among participants. When sharing with the entire group, it is imperative to talk about what kinds of insight you gained through this life story meditation without referring to personal information. By sharing, you can learn about others' experiences of Insight meditation and use them as references for your own meditation practice. When you practice this method alone, if you share your insights with a supervisor or close friend or colleague, you can prevent your meditation practice from becoming self-righteous and instead facilitate appropriate growth.

たとえば、つらい経験を思い出すことによって、自分が傷つくことになる

【展開例】

①自分にとってネガティブな体験を1つ思い出すために5分間観察する

②ネガティブな過去の出来事を1つ、15分間洞察する

③グループで実施する場合は、メンバーでシェアする

④ポジティブな過去の出来事を1つ思い出すために5分間観察する

⑤ポジティブな過去の出来事を1つ、15分間洞察する

⑥最後にメンバー内で、各15分ずつ話す人と聴く人に役割を分かれて、お互いにシェアする。

⑦全体でのシェアをする。

のではないかと考えてしまいますが、観察瞑想による客観的な洞察をすることによって、自分が苦しむことはありません。客観的な視座は、冷静な感覚の中で行うことで、感情的な主観を離れるからです。

　洞察瞑想とは、やがて、過去を手放すために、振り返りをして、やがて苦しみやそのときの辛さを手放して、忘れていく作業なのです。

　自分を一番知っているのは誰ですか。それは自分自身ですよね。だから苦しむのですが、真実を知っているのもまた、ほかでもない自分自身なのです。そして自分を1番愛せるのも自分自身です。

　このように、辛かった自分、寂しかった過去を自分で修復するプログラムが洞察瞑想であり、「愛されていなかった幼い頃の私」を発見したならば、幼児期の自分をもう1度よく思い出して「おまえもよく頑張ったね」と、今の自分が幼い時の心を抱きしめてあげましょう。その慈愛表現の作業が、自分を癒してくれます。これはSelf-Care（自己ケア）と自然治癒力になります。

　スピリチュアルケアのスーパービジョン（指導者の意見と考察）では、グループワークなどで前述の「生育歴分析」を行って、自己や他者への気づきを訓練します。こういう訓練を通じて、スピリチュアルケアの資質も高まっていきます。

　臨床瞑想法では基本的には自分1人で自己の内面世界に気づきを促すこと

To effectively practice these Observing and Insight meditations, you can place each event "on the table" in your mind as if loading data to a personal computer. In Observing Meditation, you mentally place relevant people and their relationships around you in the past situation. You can then observe your position vis-à-vis the other persons in the situation as well as your distance and intimacy with him or her in a way similar to "family systems" models.

In Insight meditation, you recall your concrete emotions and thoughts of your past. Next, you take the perspectives of other people in that situation, identify how you feel while empathizing with them, and reflect on what insights you gain as the result. You practice such a self-insight chronologically, when you were 0-5 years old, 5-10 years old, 10-15 years old, 15-20 years old, in your 20s, 30s, 40s, 50s, 60s and so on, and penetrate into the perspectives of your father, mother, brother and sister, grandparents, relatives, acquaintances, friends, and coworkers and neighbors. This practice improves your self-understanding.

People tend to think that recalling difficult experiences is painful. However, neutral observation in Observing Meditation does not distress you because the objective perspective allows you to stay calm and keep a distance from the emotional ego. This is why it is important to deepen your practice with the previous exercises first. That is, once you are able to calm your mind and see things more objectively, Insight meditation is the process through which you let go of the past events and associated suffering and pain through reflection.

Who knows you best? It's you. This is why you suffer, but it is also none other than you who knows the truth and can love yourself most deeply. Insight meditation is the program that cures us from past suffering, pain and loneliness. If you find your younger self being unloved, recall your childhood carefully and hug your younger self, saying "You did your best."

Section 3.   Four methods of meditation (Preparing for meditation practice)●65

ができるようなトレーニングを行います。さらに習得するためには、瞑想後のグループワークやシェアリングで、お互いの気づきについて話し合うことが、きわめて有効なのです。

• 心の構図を理解すると瞑想が深まる

瞑想のために、構成図を使って仏教の心理学的理解を把握し、心の探求を深めます（46ページ図10を参照）。

日常の心は、五官六根（眼、耳、鼻、舌、身、意識）によって外界を観察し、その見た現象を脳が判断して、自分の想いや思策に反映させます。唯識では眼識（視覚）・耳識（聴覚）・鼻識（嗅覚）・舌識（味覚）・身識（触覚）を前知識とし、六識にはネガティブやポジティブな感情や意思を含めたものが想念として蓄積されます。

これは基本的には脳内の作用ですが、脳の中にそういう特別な部分があるかというとそういう感覚ではなく、身体全体でとらえていく感覚と受け止めてください。

瞑想を始めるとその想念が浮かんでは消え、消えては浮かびます。初歩的な瞑想段階ではこの想念の影響を受けて、集中できないときがあります。

その想念帯は仏教心理学の唯識[6]（「六識」とマナ（末那）識、アラヤ（阿頼耶）識の八識）でマナ識に相当し煩悩といいます。したがって、とてもつらい体験をすると、一般にいうトラウマやPTSD（心的外傷後ストレス障害）などが、想念の底辺にあるマナ識に蓄積されます。

このマナ識は利己心や執着心の支配するところなので、瞑想の中でも特に重要な洞察の対象となるところです。ネガティブな思いを保持し続ける限りにおいては、なかなか自己の安心や覚醒は生まれてきません。むしろマナ識（トラウマやPTSD）の影響を受けて、つらい人生だけが続きます。

ここでブッタは、四諦八聖道などの、瞑想実践、仏道実践によって、四苦八苦からの解脱を教えています。仏教ではもう１つ深い心の世界を用意します。それがアラヤ識です。アラヤ識は心理学的には深層意識とか潜在意識などと称して、人間の心の奥底を意味する意識層で、「過去世の記憶、種の保存、

Such an expression of self-care and self-benevolence can be deeply healing in many ways.

In spiritual-care supervision, spiritual care workers practice the analysis of life history and develop awareness toward self and others through group activities. These training activities improve their abilities in providing spiritual care.

In Clinical Meditation, you basically practice how to improve the awareness of your inner self by yourself, but if you engage in group activities, sharing insights with each other, you can make progress more effectively.

- **You can deepen your meditation practice by understanding the structure of your mind.**

Understanding Buddhist psychology with the help of such structures that map the mind (see p.46 fig.10) can deepen your meditation practice. In Buddhism, the ordinary mind observes the world around you using eyes, ears, nose, tongue, body (five sense organs) and thoughts or consciousness (what Buddhist teachings call the sixth sense organ). All of these together are called Gokan rokkon 五官六根, and the brain judges what it perceived and reflects through its thoughts and considerations. In Yogacara Buddhist thought (yuishiki 唯識), the five senses of vision, audition, olfaction, taste, and touch belong to intrinsic knowledges, and positive and negative emotions and feelings as the earlier discussed Sōnen are accumulated in the sixth sense of consciousness. Please understand this composition as occurring within your whole body rather than only within your brain.

Beginners often cannot concentrate on meditation as Sōnen comes in and out of your mind. This Sōnen zone is equivalent to Manashiki of worldly desires in Yogacara of Buddhist psychology.[6]

When you have distressing experiences, traumatic memories are

Section 3.　Four methods of meditation (Preparing for meditation practice)●67

未来への提示」を司るといわれています。仏教では「大円鏡智」といいます。大円鏡智は大きく丸い円のような鏡の精神世界を表していますので、すべての真実をありのままに観察し、思量する清らかな世界を意味します。

　弘法大師空海の伝えた密教では、アラヤ識の奥に九識としてアマラ（阿摩羅）識、十識として「秘密荘厳心」を構築して、宇宙意識とつながる曼荼羅世界の深遠なる世界を瞑想的に導いています。

　洞察瞑想をする目的は、悩みという自我状態を単に避け続けたり、逃避したりする解決法ではなく、煩悩を直視して、生きようとする人間力を養うことにあります。最初は自己防衛が働き、ネガティブな感情や意思を見ないようにする感覚が生じます。しかしそれも自己洞察瞑想のプロセスなので、自己卑下することなく、丁寧に自分とかかわることです。客観的な自己洞察でそういう自分をも許して、やがて安らかな心境が生まれてきます。

　洞察瞑想の目標は、想念を突き抜け、マナ識も突き抜けて、アラヤ識という安寧の境地を獲得することなのです。心理学的にはそのような意識の変容を「変性意識状態」（altered state of consciousness）といいます。

　仏教の瞑想は、初期のシャマタ、ヴィパッサナーなどを修練し、後世にはさまざまな方法論をもつ密教瞑想を習得して、悟りを目的とした深い洞察瞑想や瑜伽行を積み重ねてきたのです。

3）たかめる瞑想（生成、促進瞑想法）

　「たかめる」とは、自分の中にある、生きようとする力や心身の機能を高めることです。

　インドでは、丹田（臍の下にあたる部分）にある生命エネルギーを高める方法が、ヨーガの瞑想法にあり、その後の仏教にも影響を与えました。中国では、気功や道教に用いられて不老長寿の志向が盛んになり、また密教の瞑想にも応用され、月輪観（自心に満月のような丸いこころを描くこと）、光明瞑想などに発展しました。

　ヨーガの経典には、心身の感覚のバランスをはかり、より次元の高い境地、

accumulated in Manashiki at the depths of Sōnen. This Manashiki possesses selfishness and attachment, which is an important object of Insight meditation. As long as you have negative emotions, peace of mind and awakening do not occur; rather, your suffering continues due to such stresses in the Manashiki (e.g., trauma and post-traumatic stress disorder).

The Buddha explained emancipation from sets he called the four and eight kinds of suffering (the four sufferings, mentioned earlier are: birth, old age, sickness, and death; the eight sufferings are those four, plus: parting from loved ones, meeting disliked ones, not getting what one seeks, and suffering related to aspects of being known as the skandhas). He taught that emancipation from suffering occurs by means of meditation practice and through Buddhist teachings of the Four Noble Truths and the fourth truth known as the Eightfold Path (see p.19,21). Buddhism also describes a deep layer of mind called "Arayashiki." Arayashiki refers to a deep part of mind which corresponds in some ways to the unconsciousness or subconsciousness in psychology. Although it also includes an aspect called "Daienkyōchi 大円鏡智," which is like a pure spiritual world with a round mirror shape, reflecting all truths as they really are.

Esoteric Buddhism as explained by Kukai suggests that meditation practice leads people to the deep world of the universal consciousness.

The aim of Insight meditation is not to avoid suffering caused by the ego but to confront worldly desires directly and develop the power to live more fully as a human being. At the first stage of meditation practice, most people turn away from negative emotions or thoughts because of the instinct of self-defense. However, it is part of the process of Insight meditation, and you need to carefully communicate with yourself without yielding to self-hatred. You can forgive yourself through Insight meditation and reach states of calmness. That is, the aim of Insight meditation is to break through Sōnen and Manashiki, attaining Arayashiki

Section 3. Four methods of meditation (Preparing for meditation practice)●69

本当の我（プルシャ＝真我）に到達する方法が詳しく説かれています。ヨーガの瞑想法は、長い伝統の中で培われた叡智が存在し、そのエネルギーの活用法は仏教、密教に受け継がれています。密教は、チベット仏教が有名ですが、日本では比叡山の天台密教と高野山の真言密教があります。編者はその高野山で密教瞑想の修行をしました。

　たかめる瞑想にはエネルギーレベルや免疫力を上げ、病気になるのを防ぐといった効果があります。また、これまでの研究から、瞑想によって心身の機能がアップすることも解明されてきました。

　具体的には、心拍数の安定・血圧の降下、脳や心臓への血流の増加、脳波・筋電信号・皮膚抵抗の正の変化、睡眠や消化の良好化、イライラ感の減少、病気の頻度や期間の減少、仕事中の事故やロスの減少、人間関係の改善、自己実現、感情・スピリチュアル指数の向上などです。また、アレルギー性疾患、ぜんそく、消化性疾患、がん、心臓疾患、不安、うつ（神経症）、糖尿病、高血圧、過敏性腸症候群、薬物依存（喫煙、アルコールも含む）、片頭痛、緊張型頭痛等の治癒および改善がみられるという報告もあります。（大下大圓、『瞑想療法』医学書院、2010）

　編者は和歌山県立医科大学の附属病院などで、脳神経内科教授のもとで科学研究費に採用された「軽度認知症の瞑想応用」の生理学的、精神医学的研究をしました。その結果、軽度認知症の患者や家族が瞑想で「気分が好転した」ことが明らかになりました。この生理学的研究報告成果は2023年「第42回日本認知症学会学術集会」で「軽度認知症者を対象としたゆるめる瞑想の効果」として、「軽度認知症者のエネルギー覚醒は上昇し、コルチゾールとアドレナリンが有意に低下し、生理的なストレス指標の軽減効果を確認した」と報告されました。

　またB大学医科学研究所などの共同研究者で、心拍計や脳血流を測定する機器（機能的近赤外分光法：fNIRS）をつかって、臨床瞑想法の4つの段階を順に測定をしました。これらの結果からも瞑想の段階的変化を生理学的に確認することができました。現在最終分析に入っていますが、得られたデータからは「たかめる瞑想、ゆだねる瞑想」は、「ゆるめる瞑想、みつめる瞑想」

as the state of peace. This is called an "altered state of consciousness" in psychology.

Meditation in Buddhism has incorporated the trainings of Shamata and Vipassanā as well as various methods of Esoteric Buddhism, consolidating deep Insight meditation for the purpose of Enlightenment.

3) "Energizing Meditation" (creation/reverence)

What is energized in "Energizing Meditation" is the power of your own life and your mental and physical functions.

Yoga meditation in India invented a method of elevating vital energy in the Tanden (丹田, a point in the body, just below the navel) and later influenced Buddhism and various teachings. Qigong and Taoism in China incorporated the method in their own pursuits of Immortality. Meditation in Esoteric Buddhism also applied it to Moon Disk meditation (Gachirinkan 月輪観) in which you visualize a pure and faultless full moon in your mind, as well as Radiance meditation.

The yoga scriptures provide a detailed explanation of how to attain a higher state of mind and true self (Purusa) by improving the balance of body and mind. These yoga meditations have accumulated wisdom regarding how to use energy, which were then inherited by Buddhism and Esoteric Buddhism in particular.

Some studies have shown that Energizing Meditation may help enhance physical and mental functions, improve the levels of energy and immunity, and prevent disease. Specifically, meditation may also help stabilize heart rates, lower blood pressure, increase blood flow to heart and brain, normalize brain waves, myoelectric signal and resistivity of skin, improve sleep quality and digestion, reduce irritation, decrease disease frequency, shorten periods of illness, reduce accidents at work, attain self-actualization,

とは異なった脳や心拍の動きがありました。これらの結果から、瞑想方法の違いによって自律神経やホルモン系に対する異なる影響があることが示唆されます。

• たかめる瞑想の方向性

　たかめる瞑想は、イメージなどを積極的に活用した瞑想で、ゆるめる瞑想、みつめる瞑想の延長にあります。瞑想時のゆったりした呼吸は、自律神経の1つである副交感神経を優位にし、それが血管へ作用した結果、動脈壁はより伸びやかで弾力性に富むようになり、血液は、末梢抵抗に遭遇しながらも内臓の器官や組織にスムーズに運ばれます。脳の活動と筋肉の緊張は抑えられ、血液が体内のシステムを上手に循環することによって、心身の機能は向上し、健康状態も向上するのです。

　実際に、瞑想が脳や筋肉に好転的な影響を与えて、健康生成に大きな貢献をしていることは、さまざまな研究から解明されています。健康生成論とは、私たちが健康を増進するうえで助けとなる力のことです。健康生成論は後述します。

　さらに、現代の精神科医療にも瞑想は取り入れられ、薬物療法だけでない新しい精神療法としての領域を担っています。我が国でも、統合医療の研究やネットワーク活動が盛んになり、エビデンス（医療的根拠）を中心に展開される西洋医学と、人の全体像を診る東洋医学との統合や連携が起きています。これは心身統合論でもあり、生と死を統合的にみる「心身一如」の生き方なのです。

　私は、近隣のＡ精神科病院のデイケアにおいて、うつ病やパニック障害の患者さんを中心に臨床瞑想法を実施したことがあります。また別の医療機関では、がん末期、慢性疾患の方に臨床瞑想法を施して、心身機能の向上に活用されています。

　また、たかめる瞑想は自らの自然治癒力を向上させます。瞑想を健全的に活用することによって自らの心身をコントロールし、日々の健康に役立て、安らかな心境に至ることができるのです。つまり「たかめる」とは、身体レ

improve interpersonal relationships and the emotion and spirituality index, and so on. According to some studies, meditation also alleviates and cures asthma, hyperacidity, cancer, heart disease, anxiety, distress, diabetes, high blood pressure, irritable colitis, drug dependence, addiction to alcohol and smoking and migraine headaches (大下大圓Oshita Daien. (2010). *瞑想療法 Meisō ryōhō*, 医学書院 Igakushoin).

We examined physiological and psychiatric effects of meditation on patients with mild cognitive impairment (MCI) and their family members as part of the Grants-in-aid for Scientific Research led by a professor of neurology at Wakayama Prefectural Medical University. The results showed that patients and family members felt better due to meditation: the energy arousal score significantly increased and cortisol and adrenaline significantly decreased in MCI patients. We presented the results at the 42nd Annual Meeting of the Japan Society for Dementia Research. In another study, we collaborated with researchers at the Medical University Faculty of Medicine and other institutions to measure heart rates and blood flow of brain by using near-infrared spectroscopy in each stage of four meditations (Loosening Meditation, Observing Meditation, Energizing Meditation and Unifying Meditation). We found gradual changes across the four meditations. Specifically, Energizing Meditation has a different effect on brain waves and heart rates than Loosening Meditation and Observing Meditation. This implies that the different types of meditation have different effects on autonomic nervous systems and hormone secretion.

• **The trajectory of Energizing Meditation**

Energizing Meditation actively makes use of images, it is an extension of Loosening Meditation and Observing Meditation. Slow breaths during meditation activate the parasympathetic nervous system,

ベルだけではなく「どのように生きるか」「この世での使命と目的を探求する」といういようなスピリチュアルな側面の向上にも寄与します。

「たかめる瞑想」の基本は、まずしっかり呼吸すること。次に洞察瞑想で得られた心身の調整を、意図的に高めるようなイメージをつくります。このイメージが大事なのです。

ユング心理学には、個我意識から集合意識に向かう発展過程において、仏やマンダラなどの統合的な意識を瞑想によってイメージする手段として、「能動的想像（Active Imagination）」があります。能動的想像とは、「心中に起こってくる夢や観念などのイメージを抑圧することなく、能動的にはたらかせながら具体化していく方法」で、それはやがて箱庭療法、描画、アートセラピーに応用されます。

はじめはイメージをすることが苦手の方もあるかもしれませんが、幼いときに経験した風景などを思い浮かべる訓練から行うといいでしょう。

• チャクラと五大を高める

密教では身体と心を五大と識大で説明します。つまり人間の身体は５つのエネルギーでできています。それを五大といって身体を五相のエネルギーで構成しているのです。地大、水大、火大、風大、空大です。（日本の真言密教を建てた弘法大師空海は、五大の上に「識」を加えて「六大」としました。）この五大は人体に当てはめた五輪塔と同じ意味をもち、インド伝来の梵字では「ア（地）、バ（水）、ラ（火）、カ（風）、キャ（空）」と表します。

この五相に５つの音を割り当てて、音階的に「ア」という音を出してみます。低い音の「ア」（地）」を出しながら、順に音階を上げて、「キャ（空）」を出していきます。音階は、瞑想する人の出せる音で適宜に決めて実施します。

１つの音を出す訓練を繰り返した後は、それにウェーブ（声による波）を、ゆったりしたリズムから、細かいリズムへと変化させて発声します。

臨床瞑想法をグループで実習する機会があれば、２～３人が１班となり、順番に「AUM（唵）」を発声して、全体の高まりを感じ合うことも有用です。

20ページに書いたように、ヨーガや密教では体内の５つのチャクラ（下腹

which makes blood vessels more supple and allows blood to flow smoothly into internal organs and cells. Because, as mentioned before, brain activities and muscular tensions are eased, blood circulates well within the body, improving physical and mental functions and health conditions.

Meditation has been adopted by modern psychiatric medicine as one kind of new treatment apart from pharmacotherapy. Today in Japan, studies and networks of integrative medicine are growing to coordinate and synthesize evidence-based Western medicine with Eastern medicine that treats body and mind holistically. This is "Shin shin ichi nyo 心身一 如 (mind-body unity)" in Buddhism. I practiced applying Clinical Meditation to clients with depression and panic disorders at a local hospital. Clinical Meditation is also practiced with clients with terminal cancer and chronic disease at another hospital to improve their mental and physical functioning.

Energizing Meditation also enhances the power to heal. You can manage your mind and body with the use of meditation to become healthy and calm in your daily life. Energizing Meditation contributes to improving not only body functions but also spirituality in terms of reflecting on how to live and exploring your mission and purpose in this life.

To breathe in and out properly is the foundation of Elevating meditation. Next, you intentionally create an image of elevating the quality of your body and mind that was generated by Insight meditation. This kind of ability to imagine is essential.

Jungian psychology advocates "Active Imagination" as a means to imagine integrated consciousness that is associated with the Buddha and Mandala in Buddhism to help individual consciousness advance toward collective consciousness. Active imagination means actively putting dreams or ideas occurring in your mind into a concrete shape without suppressing

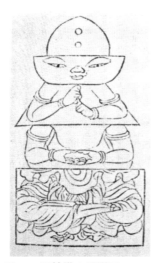

図12(fig.12)　五輪塔の原型図
An original pattern of Five-part gravestone

部、胃腸、心臓・肺、首・顔、頭頂）に地水火風空が対応するとしています。これらの発声訓練は、自己の体内にチャクラ（意識のツボ）を意識化し、五大のエネルギーを高めることを可能にするものです。

　これは近代健康医学に基づく健康生成論と符合します。健康生成（Salutogenesis）はラテン語のsalus（健康）とギリシャ語のgenesis（生成）から成る概念で、個人が健康を増進するうえで助けとなる力についてのことです。この健康生成の概念は、アントノフスキー（Aaron Antonovsky）の発表したSense of coherence＝SOC（首尾一貫感覚）に受け継がれます。

　SOC（首尾一貫感覚）は①自分の状況が理解できる（把握可能感；sense of comprehensibility）、②何とかやっていける（処理可能感；sense of manageability）、③やりがいや生きる意味が感じられる（有意味感；sense of meaningfulness）の3点が感覚を形づくっているとされます。

　たかめる瞑想をすることで身体的には脳波や自律神経、免疫系にはたらきかけて、健康回復に大きな影響を与えるばかりでなく、精神的、スピリチュアリティな向上に影響を与えSOCが向上します。

　結論的には、たかめる瞑想を実践することで、SOCが高まり、身体機能のみならず人格やスピリチュアリティの向上をはかることが可能となるのです。

them. This is also applied in sand play therapy, drawing therapy and art therapy. You may not be good at imagining at first. If so, you can begin by imagining scenes that you saw during your childhood.

- **Energizing Chakra and Godai**

According to Esoteric Buddhism, a human body consists of Godai 五大 energy (five great elements), earth, water, fire, wind and space. These five great elements correspond to a five-part gravestone found in Japan, which has five different shapes stacked one on top of the other, representing each of those elements. (see fig.12) The elements also each represent a different type of vibration or tune and allocate Sanskrit characters as sounds that accord to each vibration. The sounds, respectively, are "ah" for earth, "ba" for water, "ra" for fire, "ka" for wind, and "kya" for space or ether. You utter "a" in a lower pitch and raise the pitches step by step. At last, you utter "kya (梵字の空)" in the highest pitch. You can decide intervals as you see fit. After you practice uttering each pitch, you continuously raise and lower the pitch for each character and change the rhythm of voice from slow "ahhhh, ahhhh," to a fast "ah", "ah". It is helpful to practice this as a group, in which groups of two or three participants take turns uttering "AUM" while feeling heightened stimulation.

As described on page 21, Esoteric Buddhism sees the five elements of the human body (lower abdomen, stomach, heart and lung, neck and face, head top) corresponding to the five elements of the universe or the Chakras in yoga philosophy, associated with earth, water, fire, wind, and space, respectively. So, Esoteric Buddhism holds that such voice training enables the Chakra energy centers in your body to be awakened and the five element energies to increase. Esoteric Buddhism's founder in Japan, Kukai, added an additional energy, Shikidai (Consciousness) to the five-element system, positing six great elements.

・具体的なたかめる瞑想法の例

①声の瞑想

　自分から声を出して、身体に振動する波動を感じる瞑想

　アー、エー、イー、オー、ウーなど連続して発生をしたり、音程を変えたりしてその響きを感じる。仏教に声明（お経に曲がついている）で使用する「一越（レ）、平調（ミ）、双調（ソ）、黄鐘（ラ）、盤渉（シ）」を体の五体（下腹部、胃腸、心臓・肺、首・顔、頭頂）に合わせて声を出し、その波動の余韻を大事にしつつ、その後に瞑想をする。

②光明（ローソクやLEDランプなど）を使った瞑想

　床に燭台にのったローソクの灯を見つめながら瞑想する。その灯りが自分に入ってくる、自分が灯りに入っていくようなイメージの瞑想をする。

③大きな炎（焚火や仏教の護摩行など）を見ながら瞑想

　この時に真言（マントラ）を唱えながら見つめたあとに、瞑想をする。

④森の中や樹々の根本での瞑想

　大きな木の根元で、その木の生命を感じながら瞑想をする。

　深い森の中で、大自然に抱かれていることを感じながら瞑想をする。

⑤滝、川での瞑想

　大きな川のほとりや、滝の近くでその精妙な気を感じながら瞑想をする

⑥山岳での瞑想

　山の頂上や中腹の景色の良いところで雄大な自然を感じながら瞑想する。

⑦海洋での瞑想

　浜辺や船にのって、大海原を見ながら瞑想をする。

４）ゆだねる瞑想法（統合、融合瞑想法）

　「ゆだねる」とは、自分の「いのち」を「大いなるいのち」や「偉大なるいのち」に委ねることです。

　「自分の命を委ねるなんて、そんな恐ろしいことはできません」という人は多いと思います。しかしこれは、あえていえば「人事を尽くして天命を待

This converges with the concept of Salutogenesis in modern medicine. Salutogenesis is a coined word comprised of "salus (health)" in Latin and "genese (generation)" in Greek and means the power to be healthier. Salutogenesis was later elaborated in the concept of Sense of Coherence (SOC) by Aaron Antonovsky. The Sense of Coherence consists of three elements: Sense of Comprehensibility (feeling able to understand one's situation), Sense of Manageability (feeling able to get by) and Sense of meaningfulness (feeling fulfilled and that there is meaning in life). (Antonovsky A. *Unraveling the Mystery of Health*. 1987. San Francisco: Jossey-Bass Inc.).

Energizing Meditation engages brain waves, autonomic nervous system and immune systems, generating significant effects on health recovery, and addresses improving one's mind, spirituality, and Sense of Coherence (SOC). In conclusion, practicing Energizing Meditation improves SOC, enhancing not only physical function but I also believe elements of one's personality and spirituality as well.

- **Concrete examples of "Energizing Meditation"**

① Vocal meditation: Meditation while feeling the vibration of your voice in your body

You feel the vibration of your own voice when making sounds, changing pitches of "ah", "eh", "eee", "oh", "oo". You make each sound corresponding to each body element: lower abdomen, stomach, heart and lung, neck and face, and top of the head, respectively. After feeling the vibration of your own voice, you meditate.

② Meditation with the radiance of a candle or LED light

You meditate while watching the radiance of a candle. You imagine that the radiance comes into your body and your body into the radiance while meditating.

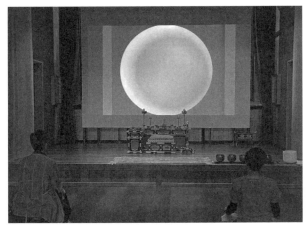

図13（fig.13）　光の瞑想
Light Meditation

つ」という心境です。たとえば、自分では努力や学びをせずに幸せが棚ぼた式に手に入るように願って、ことの成り行きを見守っている姿勢とは真逆にあるものです。

　ゆだねるのは仏、神、天、宇宙、自然、先祖などの大いなる世界で、そのことを「サムシンググレイト（何か偉大なるもの）」と表現する人もいます。小さな我執にとらわれるのでなく、自己や他者を超えた大きな世界に思いを馳せ、その仏教でいう「大我(たいが)」に生きる価値を見つけるという意識であり、覚悟です。

　現在の意識状態を確認してから、それが次第に変容していく様を客観的に観察し続けることです。ゆだねる瞑想とは、心が幸福感と安らぎ感に満たされ、大いなる命と融合している感覚が長時間にわたって継続している状態です。

　これまで私は、個人と全体性の健康に関する概念を、マンダラの思考や東洋的な叡智を探りながら解釈を試みてきましたが、本書で繰り返し述べていることは、瞑想は心身の全体的な健康生成に有効であるということです。

③ Meditation with a large flame of a bonfire

After watching a large flame while also possibly chanting a Mantra, you meditate.

④ Meditation in a forest and at the foot of a tree

You meditate at the foot of a tree while imagining you feel the tree's life. You meditate in a deep forest while feeling embraced by nature.

⑤ Meditation near a waterfall or river

You meditate near a waterfall or a river while imagining you feel its subtle energy.

⑥ Meditation on a mountain

You meditate at the top or on the side of a mountain with beautiful scenery while feeling embraced by the magnificence of nature around you.

⑦ Meditation by the sea

You meditate on the beach or on a boat in the sea while watching the open sea.

4) "Unifying Meditation" (integration/unification)

"Unifying Meditation" aims at unifying one's own life into "Something Greater". Many people might think that it is awful to surrender their own lives. Actually, it means "doing your best and entrusting everything to the universe". It is the opposite attitude of hoping for happiness without making effort or learning. You imagine or feel yourself unifying with the existence around you, which some people call "Something Greater". Allowing yourself to be a part of "Something Greater" means making up your mind to contemplate the transcendent world without distinguishing oneself from others and finding the value in letting go of egotism and attachment to the world of desires.

・ゆだねる瞑想の具体的な方法

ゆだねるというイメージがわかりにくい方は、外のエネルギーとの交流や融合を身近な道具を使って、瞑想に活かすこともできます。

(a) 前出の大日如来の宇宙性を表す「阿字観」「月輪観」の本尊を使用することも有効ですが、それらが身近に無い場合は、ローソクの燈明を利用するといいでしょう。仏壇や神棚があるお宅ならローソク立てがあると思います。または、100円ショップなどで小さなローソク立てと5〜8センチくらいのローソクを準備してください。

　室内を暗くして、火を灯したローソクが少し強調されるような雰囲気を演出します。次に、そのローソクを目の高さになるように台の上に乗せます。目の高さより高くならないように気をつけてください。

　そして、ゆるめる瞑想で心身をニュートラルにしたうえで、ローソクの灯りを見続けます。灯りを見続ける時間は3〜5分が適当でしょう。やがて、「灯りが自分の中に入ってくる」「自分がローソクに入っていく」というような「入我我入観」ができるようになります。対象と自己との融合的な感覚が生まれてきます。

(b) 滝や山を見て

　臨床瞑想法をトレーニングするときに、近くに大自然があれば、積極的に利用しましょう。拙著『ケアと対人援助に活かす瞑想療法』（医学書院）では、自然界での瞑想法で、樹木瞑想、山岳瞑想、滝川瞑想などを紹介していますが、大自然のエネルギーは人間力を越えたものです。

　大木が茂る森林の中では、新鮮な空気を身体いっぱい吸い込んで気持ちのよい瞑想ができます。また勢いよく滝つぼに落ちる滝を前にして瞑想すると、その水のエネルギーによる浄化的感覚がカタルシスを生み出します。清らかな意識に充たされると、自己の存在がいとおしくなり、あらゆることに感謝の念さえ浮かぶのです。

　無理にそのように思わなくても、滝が流れ落ちるときのエネルギーからは、自己を超えて躍動する自然界のパワーをそのまま感じ取ることができ

In this Unifying Meditation, you observe your state of consciousness and keep observing how it changes over time. Unifying Meditation creates the state of happiness, calmness and a long-lasting sense of being unified with the surrounding existence.

So far I have tried to explain concepts that are related to individual and collective health by using Mandala and Eastern wisdom. Essentially, I want to suggest that meditation is useful for holistically strengthening mental and physical health.

- **Concrete examples of "Unifying Meditation"**

If you have difficulty imagining what it means to unify, you can interact and integrate with external energies with the help of familiar objects.

(a) You can use an image of the "A" syllable or the circle of light described above, which symbolizes the light and goodness of the universe. If you do not have it handy, you may use the radiance of a candle. Please prepare a candle about 5-8 centimeters long with a candle holder, or another type of candle that will last long enough through your meditation period.

Make the room dark to slightly emphasize the radiance of a candle. Next, place the candle at about eye level. Be careful not to place it above the eye level.

After you practice Loosening Meditation, you keep watching the radiance of a candle for 3-5 minutes. Then, try to start feeling a sense of "the radiance coming into me" and "I am going into radiance". This is called "Nyuga ganyu kan 入我我入観". It is the sense of unification between oneself and an object.

(b) For Clinical Meditation training, one may use nearby nature. As I illustrated some nature meditations with trees, mountains and rivers and waterfalls above and in my book *Clinical Meditation for*

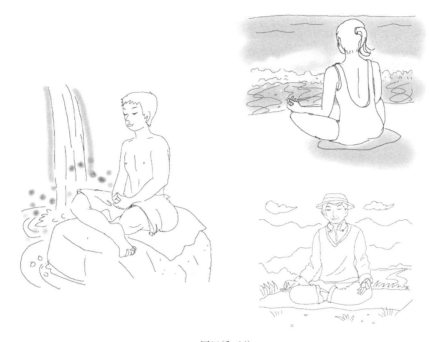

図14（fig.14）

ます。これも変性意識です。

　瞑想法としては、最初はその流れる滝を見続けます。やはり3〜5分間の凝視をしながら、「滝のエネルギーが自分に入ってくる」と意識します。

　次に「自分のすべてが滝に入っていく」とイメージし、瞑想に入ります。これも15〜30分くらいの丁寧な瞑想をします。こうして、さまざまな場所でゆだねる瞑想を応用できます。

・神・仏（法縁）と融合

　「法縁」仏教の法（ダルマ）とは宇宙意識とのつながりのことを言います。一神教の文化圏では「大いなるもの」（サムシンググレイト）や「神」の意識

Interpersonal Care and Support, the energy of nature surpasses human power.

You can meditate comfortably under a big tree in a forest by fully inhaling fresh air. When you meditate in front of a waterfall creating powerful splashes, water energy creates the feeling of purification, leading to catharsis. If you are filled with a sense of pure consciousness, you will cherish yourself and even feel grateful for everything under the sun. You do not have to force yourself to think so. From the energy of the waterfall, you can naturally feel the power of nature transcending an individual self. This, too, is an altered state of consciousness.

To practice such meditation, you first keep watching a waterfall, as you do with the radiance of a candle. You keep watching the waterfall for 3-5 minutes by visualizing its energy coming into you. Next, imagine your entire self going into the waterfall and meditate for 15-30 minutes wholeheartedly. Thus, you can practice Unifying Meditation at various places.

• **Unification**

The scope of Unifying Meditation is as wide and deep as that of Energizing Meditation, and the practice of Unifying Meditation is obviously connected with how much a practitioner explores spirituality and its thought to be important to practice regularly to enhance spirituality.

In Buddhist spirituality, filling your heart with the four Brahmavihara virtues, compassion, and love to maintain peace of mind and imagine vast universal consciousness is a goal to be cultivated. Specifically, the four virtues consist of Ji 慈 (a heart of wishing and caring about others' happiness), Hi 悲 (a heart of compassion to alleviate others' suffering), Ki 喜(a

とつながることを指します。

　自己を包摂する宇宙意識や曼荼羅の仏、菩薩と融合するためには、専門的な訓練が必要です。ただし、一般在家の人であっても、融合の意識構造を理解できれば、心が幸福感とやすらぎに満たされ、大いなる命と融合している感覚が長時間にわたって継続している状態を達成することは可能であるといえます。

　それには、日頃から自己を超える意識（トランスパーソナル）に関心をもつことと、常に自己を客観視する瞑想の鍛錬が必須です。

　臨床瞑想法指導者養成講習会などでも、その要素を訓練しますが、まずはイメージする訓練が大事です。曼荼羅や仏、菩薩の画像などを日頃から観ておくことも有用でしょう。

　自分が「大いなるもの」を想定しておいて、瞑想に入ってからそのエネルギーを意識することが大事です。セミナーでは前述のローソクの灯りや、曼荼羅を用いて訓練します。また法縁の中に、己とつながっている先祖の意識をイメージして、先に亡くなった肉身との和合や和解を達成する人もいます。

　ゆだねる瞑想の領域は、たかめる瞑想とともにその範疇は広くて深いものがありますから、その人のスピリチュアリティの探求と連動していることが明らかです。日頃から自己のスピリチュアリティをたかめる訓練が重要といえます。

　日ごろから「慈・悲・喜・捨」（四無量心）という「慈悲と愛」の心を充足して、平和な心を呼び起こし、宇宙的な広大な意識を日ごろからイメージすることも大事です。具体的には「慈：相手の幸せを望み慈しむ心」「悲：苦しみを救ってあげようとする憐れみの心」「喜：相手の幸せを直に喜べる心」「捨：平和な心で、執着を手放す心」という精神性を柱として瞑想生活をすることです。

　世界のどこでも飢餓、貧困、紛争や国家間の戦争は絶えないのですが、常に平和を希求するこころを失ってはいけません。

heart of sincerely congratulating others' happiness) and Sha 捨 (a heart of peacefully releasing attachments). Hunger, poverty, and conflicts and wars between nations persist in the world, but we must not lose the spirit of seeking peace.

Section 3. Four methods of meditation (Preparing for meditation practice)●87

第4章

対人援助のための臨床瞑想法のトレーニング

1）実施手順

　対人援助のための臨床瞑想法の実践については、すでに臨床瞑想法の構成については前述しました。あなたが、主催者として実際に、クライアントに対して臨床瞑想を行う前に、対人援助の方法として「構造的臨床瞑想法」「非構造的臨床瞑想法」「半構造的臨床瞑想法」のどれを採用するかを最初に決めておく必要があります。

　「構造的瞑想療法」とは、明確な瞑想療法のプログラムを立てて、その評価や成果まで予測して実習の流れや瞑想をリードする人とクライアントとの位置関係も事前に計画することです。その実習にあたっては、場所の選定、時間の制約、セッションの流れなどを他の援助スタッフと事前の打ち合わせをして、予想される成果や実習後の効果についての検証も必要です。これは、特に個人の成長の記録や療養経緯を客観的に説明していくことで互いの共通理解とセッションの深まりを達成するうえで有効です。また他の心身状態を改善するアプローチと併用して実践することにおいても、くわしい記録は振りかえりや次回へのアプローチをすることに役立ちます。

　「非構造的瞑想療法」とは、事前の綿密なクライアントの情報などの分析はなくても、その場で簡略化したアセスメントを行い、やや即興的に瞑想療法を行うことです。このセッションには自由性があり、特に場所も特定せずに、クライアントの自由な思いを尊重して、瞑想活動を行うことです。この療法は、セラピストの十分な経験が必要とされます。

　「半構造的瞑想療法」は前述の2つを併合する形で、場所や時間にあまりとらわれないで、クライアントの自由な瞑想意欲を尊重して、適宜に行うも

88●第4章　対人援助のための臨床瞑想法のトレーニング

Section 4.

How Clinical Meditation for Interpersonal Support is practiced in the Japanese Cultural Context

1) Implementation procedures

Thus far, I briefly introduced the practice and structure of Clinical Meditation and its use for interpersonal support.

Yet, before you actually apply Clinical Meditation to support clients, you have to decide between one of its three application models of structured, semi-structured or non-structured.

Structured Clinical Meditation means that the organizers strictly plan the flow of the session, the positional dynamics between leader and client, location, time constraints and so on, while making arrangements with other staff for care related to predicted outcomes. After the session, the organizers need to verify the effects of the meditation session. Objective record of client growth and recuperation during the process is very useful to be able to share that experience and help the Clinical Meditation become more effective from session to session. Detailed records are helpful when combining it with another therapy for improving their body and mind or reviewing and preparing for the next approach.

Non-structured Clinical Meditation refers to guiding the client in meditation after basic assessment without prior analysis of information

のでありますが、かならず実習後にその記録をとって、個人の情報として大切に施設などで保管することです。これは当然のことですが、データは個人情報にあたりますから、その管理には一般カルテとおなじような守秘義務の扱いとなります。

　次に、臨床瞑想法を行う際の具体的な流れについて確認しておきましょう。前に述べた「ゆるめる瞑想」「みつめる瞑想」「たかめる瞑想」「ゆだねる瞑想」の理解のもとに、臨床瞑想法を実施するための準備とその具体的な方法を説明します。

　まず、臨床瞑想法を実践しようとする対象（クライアント）のアセスメントを行います。クライアントがどのような気持ちでいるのか、今の感情や意思はどうかなどを、主に聞き取りやアセスメントシートなどを使用して確認します。セラピストが心得ておかねばならないことは次の5点です。

● **セラピストの心得**

①ケアのニーズに対する気づきをすること。

　（臨床瞑想法が必要であるかどうかの確認）

②セラピストが状況を改善する方法についての知識をもつこと。

　（臨床瞑想法によって、少なくともクライアントの心身に改善が期待されること）

③セラピストが援助しようとする意思をもつこと。

　（セラピストが明確な援助意識をもつこと）

④実践方法を選択し、実施すること。

　（4つのメソッドから選択する）

⑤クライアントの変化は、ほかの人やほかの状況にとって好ましいものではなくても、クライアントにとって好ましいものに基づくこと。

　（指導者の自己満足に終わらないように、対象者のスピリチュアリティに焦点をあてること）

　これらは、ケアやコミュニケーションの場面でどのように瞑想を展開していくべきか、セラピストの資質にかかわることでもありますから、日頃から

about them or planning for a particular place. The therapist can deal flexibly with a client's request at the moment in the session. However, a therapist must have enough experience to practice meditation within such circumstances.

Semi-structured Clinical Meditation comes between the aforementioned Structured and Non-structured formats. Time and place are not restricted in this type of session and the therapist provides meditation while respecting a client's requests.

Following are concrete steps for preparation and practical ways to provide Clinical Meditation while determining whether to guide "Loosening Meditation", "Observing Meditation", "Energizing Meditation" and/or "Unifying Meditation" as described above.

At first, you assess how the client is feeling, keeping record of their emotions and intentions in your assessment.

- **There are five points which therapists should first pay attention to:**
① Be aware of the client's needs, (especially, in this case, whether Clinical Meditation is needed or not).
② Have proper knowledge to address a client's condition (the clear intention for somehow improving a client's physical and mental state by providing Clinical Meditation).
③ Maintain your intention to help the client (a firm intention of support).
④ Select the most beneficial of the four methods and provide it.
⑤ Keep in mind and heart that any change is focused on what is best for the client not for other people (focusing on the client's sense of well-being and not on one's own self-satisfaction).

Keeping these five points in mind helps maintain a mental state of care

心がけておくことが大切です。

　臨床瞑想法を提供しようとする側には、クライアントの身体的・精神的なニーズを把握し、スピリチュアルな局面を的確に観察する力が求められます。さらには、臨床瞑想法を提供する側とされる側が対立的構造ではなく、互いに理解し、双方のスピリチュアリティに基点をおいた深いかかわりをもつことが重要です。

　臨床瞑想法をスピリチュアルケアの一環として行う場合は、縁の関係性を肯定的に受け入れ、クライアントのスピリチュアルな領域のニーズや苦悩を全人格的に受容、把握し、注意深く、慎重に行うことを心がけてください。

　これらを踏まえて、臨床瞑想法を実践する際の５つのステップを提示します。

　　・臨床瞑想法を実践する際の５つのステップ
①インテーク（導入）：コミュニケーション、ニーズに対する気づきと共通理解。
②セッション（瞑想実施）：方法の選択と適宜な実践活動。
③シェアリング（分かち合い）：気づきにつながる語り合い。
④インテグラル・サポート（援助の統合性）：幸福感、新たな心身の健康生成に対するサポート。
⑤セルフチェック（検証、評価）：セッション内容の振り返りと記録

　では、臨床瞑想法における言葉かけやケア行動の一例を挙げてみましょう。

２）健常者を対象とするとき

　準備体操や姿勢を変えることに問題のない方たちを対象とするときの手順です。クライアントは、１人でも複数でも同様に進行することができます。

toward the client and ensures we are keeping our capacity to provide that care, while helping others to cultivate their states of meditation.

Providers of Clinical Meditation should maintain a strong sense and will to carefully observe and understand the client's physical and mental needs. Furthermore, it is important that providers and recipients of Clinical Meditation maintain an attitude of mutual understanding and build a deep relationship on the basis of mutual respect.

When you provide Clinical Meditation for spiritual care, you should holistically accept the client's needs and state of suffering, carefully and prudently responding to those needs.

- **I show five steps to provide Clinical Meditation as below**
① Intake: communication, awareness of needs and mutual understanding
② Session: selection of suitable method and appropriate practical activities
③ Sharing: discussion for awareness
④ Integral support: support for happiness and generating health of body and mind
⑤ Self-check: review and record the content of the session

2) When targeting healthy individuals

【Intake】
① You come to the client or group of clients with a smile.
② You briefly explain Clinical Meditation and the meditation plans for the session.
③ You ask them "Would you like to practice some meditation with me today?" If someone has any questions or uncertain issues, you earnestly answer them.

【インテーク；導入】

① 笑顔で参加者のもとへ行く。

② ひと通り瞑想の意義や方法について説明する。

③ 「もしよければ、私と一緒に瞑想をやってみませんか？」と尋ね、瞑想に対する質問や疑問などがあれば丁寧に答える。

④ 「今、どんな気分ですか、ちょっと目を閉じて自分の心に聴いてみましょう」と現在の意識の内省を促す。ここで少し静かな音楽を使用してもいい。

⑤ 「では、これから瞑想に入ります。やりたくないときは、無理をしなくていいですよ」と、了解を得たうえで安全を保証する。

⑥ 体操などを適宜活用し、姿勢や呼吸の方法を教えて、瞑想に入る。

　※瞑想のはじめと終わりに、チベッタンベル（ティンシャ）やシンギングボウルなどを使用すると脳波に共鳴して瞑想に入りやすいが、音の反応では個人差があるので注意が必要。

【セッション；瞑想】

⑦ ゆっくりと静かな口調で、瞑想の手順を伝える。

　・クライアントの一番楽な姿勢を促し、仰臥位（起きていられない人に対して寝たままでいいことを丁寧に伝える）。静座、安座（あぐらやくつろいだ座位）でもよいことを伝える。

⑧ 瞑想を行う。

　・「軽く眼を閉じてください」

　・「自分にとって気持ちが楽になるシーンをイメージしてみてください」（海、里山、花、風景など）「小さいときに遊んだ場所でもいいです」などとイメージを固定しない。

　・「口から大きく長く息を吐き、鼻から無理なくゆっくりと息を吸ってください」

　・「この呼吸を 7 回以上繰り返してみてください」または「心が落ち着くまで何度でもやってください」

　・「心の落ち着きを感じたら、あなた自身の自然な呼吸に戻してください」

④ You ask them to consider their thoughts "How do you feel?" You ask them if they would mind closing their eyes. Optionally, you can also use calming music.

⑤ If they have agreed to the meditation and you don't compel it in any way, you can say, "Now let's begin the meditation. If you don't want to do any part of this, don't worry and feel free to just rest or request that I pause or stop."

⑥ You teach the postures and how to breathe while incorporating some exercise and introduce the meditation.

＊ Most people can meditate with greater ease by using sounds of a Tibetan bell or Singing bowls at the beginning and end of a session. The sounds may be resonant with brain waves. However, consideration is needed as there are individual preferences and differences.

【Session】

⑦ Introduce clients to the meditation procedure in a slow and soft tone.

・ "You can meditate in an easy posture, sitting on a cushion or lying down is OK, if it is difficult to sit on the floor."

⑧ Start the meditation session.

・ "Please close your eyes".

・ "Please imagine a scene which helps you feel comfortable, like the sea, a village in the, mountains, flowers, or even a place where you played in your childhood". Don't be fixated on a particular image.

・ "Breathe out from the mouth full and long; breathe in from the nose comfortably and slowly."

・ "Repeat this seven times or more". Or "Repeat this till your mind feels calm".

・ "Return to a natural pace of breathing when you feel more calm."

・ "Let's go a little deeper into the meditation".

Section 4. How Clinical Meditation for Interpersonal Support is practiced in the Japanese Cultural Context●95

・「さあ瞑想に入りましょう」

※３分間以上。瞑想時間はクライアントと相談してあらかじめ決めて行うのもよいし、後半で心地よい風景などのイメージを導入してもよい。

常に本人の気持ちの安定性に配慮することが大事。

・（予定の時間になったら）「１回だけ大きく深呼吸してください」として瞑想をやめる。

・「ゆっくり背伸びをしてください。手や足を動かして、身体の感覚を取り戻してください。首を回してみましょう。どこか身体の中で違和感をもつ部分はありませんか？」

・「ハイ、これで瞑想を終わります」

【シェアリング；分かち合い】

⑨「瞑想が終わった今は、身体の感覚はどうですか？ 心はどんな気持ちですか？」とクライアントに尋ねて、セラピストがその気持ちに共感し、クライアントには、自分の気持ちや感覚を受容するよう促す。

⑩反応を聞いて、「今あなたは○○○という気持ちになっているのですね」と、その感覚や感想をペアやグループで共有したり、語り合ったりする。批判的にならないように注意すること。

【インテグラル・サポート；援助の統合性】

⑪最後に、全体的に輪になって座る。セラピストは全員の顔が確実にみえる位置に座ることが大事。顔をみて１人ひとりの発言に受け答えする。

⑫「瞑想中に何かを感じたり、気になったりしたことはありますか？」と尋ねて、その課題の意味や背景を一緒に考える。

⑬「今のあなたの気持ちは、自分を知っていくうえでとても重要なことですね。どうか、あなた自身がそのことについて今、言葉にした事実を大切にしてください」と伝える。

⑭「あなた（皆さん）と一緒に瞑想ができてよかったです。もし今後に気になることがあったら、いつでもご連絡ください」と伝え、瞑想セッションへの

＊Do the meditation for at least three minutes. You may decide the time frame with clients beforehand. You can introduce a comfortable scene towards the end. Always consider the clients' wellbeing.

· When you are ready to end the session, say "Take just one more deep breath".

· "Please feel free to stretch different parts of your body, move your arms and legs, do some neck circles, and move around a little to loosen up. If any part of you feels uncomfortable, feel free to let me know."

· "And now the Meditation session is over".

【Sharing】

⑨ "Now that the meditation is finished, take a moment to just observe how you feel? How do you feel both physically and mentally?" The therapist asks clients, empathizes with them and ask them to be accepting of what feelings and sensations arise.

⑩ You listen to a client's feedback. "So, you are feeling ○○ now". When practicing with a group of clients, feedback is shared and discussed in a group or in pairs. Pay attention not to be critical.

【Integral support】

⑪ Finally, all clients sit with the therapist in a circle. It is important for the therapist to be able to see all clients' faces. The therapist can listen and respond to each individual on a one to one basis.

⑫ You can reflect on the session as a group "What feelings or responses arose in your during the meditation session?"

⑬ You can also tell them: "Your present feelings are very important for understanding yourself. Please cherish the fact that you can put them into words".

⑭ "I am happy to meditate with you. If you have any questions, don't

参加意思を称える言葉、姿勢、態度を示して、セッションの終了を宣言する。

【セルフチェック；検証、評価】

⑮控え室に戻って、セッションについて記録し、自己評価をする。

⑯機会があれば、スタッフやスーパーバイザーと振り返りを行う。

　疑問点や改良点などスーパーバイザーの助言や指導を受けることも有効である。

3）ベッドで療養されている方への臨床瞑想法

　病気などで身体を動かしにくい方や、寝たきりの方であっても、次のように進行することができます。

【インテーク；導入】

①笑顔で病室あるいはクライアントの希望する部屋に入る。

②「今、お身体の具合などで気になることはありませんか？」「少しお話ししていいですか」と面接の了解を得る。

③「もしよければ、私と一緒に瞑想をやってみませんか？」と尋ね、瞑想に対する質問や疑問などがあれば丁寧に答える。

　※クライアントには、臥床したままでも瞑想ができることを伝える。

④部屋の空気（新鮮さ）、匂い、音などに配慮して、必要な処置をする。

　※たとえば空気がよどんでいたら、クライアントの了解を得て、新鮮な外の空気を入れるなど、場を整える。

⑤クライアントのベッドサイドに椅子などを寄せて座る。

⑥音の有無や音楽についての希望を聞いて、必要であれば、瞑想に適したものを使用する。

　※CDプレイヤーなどを事前に準備することもある。瞑想のはじめと終わりに、チベッタンベル（ティンシャ）やシンギングボウルなどを使用すると脳波に共鳴して瞑想に入りやすいが、個人差があるので確認など注意が必要。

hesitate to ask here or connect with me later". You may praise them for participation in the meditation session. You then declare the end of the session.

【Self-check】

⑮ Make note of the session and assess yourself afterwards.

⑯ You may review your session with a supervisor if it is appropriate and applicable. It is useful to receive supervision and reflect with your supervisor about any uncertainties in order to grow and improve.

3) Clinical Meditation for Clients who are sick in bed

You can proceed with a meditation session for a client who is difficult to move or bedridden.

【Intake】

① Enter the room with a kind smile for your client.

② Obtain their consent for the meeting, "Do you mind us having a chat right now? How is your body feeling at the moment?" You ask him/her "Would you like to practice meditation with me?" And if he/she has any questions or issues of uncertainty, you earnestly address them.

＊You explain that he/she can practice meditation while lying down.

③ Ask them, "Would you be interested in trying a little meditation?" Answer any questions they might have about meditation or the session you will offer.

④ Consider the space you are in with the client and any smells, noises, or air quality of the room.

＊If the air feels stale and it is within facility rules, you might ask the client's permission to open a window and let fresh air in.

Section 4.　How Clinical Meditation for Interpersonal Support is practiced in the Japanese Cultural Context●99

【セッション；瞑想】

⑦ゆっくりと静かな口調で、瞑想の手順を伝える。

・クライアントにとって一番楽な姿勢を促し、仰臥位でもベッド上の静座、安座（あぐらやくつろいだ座位）でもよいことを伝える。

⑧瞑想を行う。

・「軽く眼を閉じてください」

・「自分にとって気持ちが楽になるシーンをイメージしてみてください」（海、里山、花、風景など）「小さいときに遊んだ場所でもいいです」などとイメージを固定しない。

・「口から大きく長く息を吐き、鼻から無理なくゆっくりと息を吸ってください」

・「この呼吸を7回以上繰り返してみてください」または「心が落ち着くまで何度でもやってください」

・「心の落ち着きを感じたら、あなた自身の自然な呼吸に戻してください」

・「さあ瞑想に入りましょう」

※3分間以上。時間はクライアントと相談してあらかじめ決めて行うのもよいし、後半で心地よい風景などのイメージを導入してもよい。

常に本人の気持ちの健全性に配慮することが大事。

・（予定の時間になったら）「1回だけ大きく深呼吸してください」として瞑想をやめる。

・「ゆっくり背伸びをしてください。手や足を動かして、身体の感覚を取り戻してください。首を回してみましょう。どこか身体の中で違和感をもつ部分はありませんか？」

・「ハイ、これで瞑想を終わります」

【シェアリング；分かち合い】

⑨「瞑想が終わった今は、身体の感覚はどうですか？　どんな気分ですか？」とクライアントに尋ねて、その気持ちや感覚を受容するよう促す。

⑤ Sit in a chair near the client's bed.

⑥ Ask the client about their preferences for background music or a lack thereof. You may use appropriate meditation music if helpful.

＊As mentioned above, a Tibetan bell or Singing bowl may be helpful to begin and end the meditation session.

【Session】

⑦ You speak to a client about the steps of meditation in a slow and soft tone.

・"You can meditate in your most easy posture, lying down or a seated position on the bed". Comfort them by letting them know or reminding them that it is perfectly fine to practice the meditation while lying down just as they are.

Then follow the same procedures as p.95 ⑧.

【Sharing】

Follow the same procedures as p.97 [sharing].

【Integral support】

Also, rather than being done in a group, the reflections after the meditation are simply carried out on a one-on-one basis.

【Self-check】

The procedures described above, are of course nothing more than a model for plans which you may adapt according to the patient and facility conditions.

For example, a patient in home care may practice meditation in their own bedroom or living room. It may be easy for a patient to start

⑩反応を聞いて、「今あなたは○○○という気持ちになっているのですね」と、その感覚を共有したり、語り合ったりする。

【インテグラル・サポート；援助の統合性】

⑪「瞑想中に何かを感じたり、気になったりしたことはありますか？」と尋ねて、その課題の意味や背景を一緒に考える。

⑫今のあなたの気持ちは、自分を知っていくうえでとても重要なことですね。どうか、あなた自身がそのことについて今、言葉にした事実を大切にしてください」と伝える。

⑬「一緒に瞑想ができてよかったです。もし今後に気になることがあったら、いつでもご連絡ください」と伝えて、クライアントに共感し、応援する言葉、姿勢、態度を示す。

【セルフチェック；検証、評価】

⑭控え室に戻って、セッションについて記録し、自己評価をする。

⑮機会があれば、スタッフやスーパーバイザーと振り返りを行う。

　疑問点や改良点について、スーパーバイザーの助言、指導を受けることも有効である。

　以上の手順はあくまでも例ですから、クライアントの状況に合わせて、適宜、工夫して行ってください。

　一方、在宅ケアでは、施設のように特定の部屋やベッド上ではなく、住み慣れた自宅の一室で瞑想を行うことになります。クライアントにとっては、瞑想をやりやすい反面、あまりにも日常的な場所であるだけに、瞑想によるスピリチュアルな時空を確保するのが難しい側面もあります。

　いずれにしても、臨床瞑想法がクライアントの総合的なスピリチュアルケアに役立つように、場所や時間、周囲の環境づくりに配慮して行うことが肝心です。

　また、在宅ケアの場合は家族が同席しやすい環境にあります。家族と一緒

meditating, but still challenging to have an extraordinary experience with it. Considerations of time and place can at least help impact the quality of that experience and its overall role within holistic care. In home care, family members might also be able to readily participate in the meditation. Meditating together (a client and family members) might also be useful for alleviating family members' nursing fatigue.

4) Using Music with Clinical Meditation

Meditation can be smoothly introduced by using serene ambient music or narration sound files or video files. I am qualified as a music therapist (Gifu Pref. Music Therapist Association Certification). I often practice Clinical Meditation in combination with music therapy in temples, hospitals and even Tsunami and earthquake disaster areas like Northern Japan.

There are a lot of musical instruments at my temple, Hida-Senkōji. I often use a Tibetan bell, other kinds of bells, singing bowls, a Buddhist bell, a temple bell in practicing sessions of Clinical Meditation. I select music in accord with the wishes of patients with terminal cancer or chronic illness and provide Clinical Meditation for them using the music as back ground music (BGM). It creates special and meaningful experiences together.

I use music to help a client imagine and recall. In particular, music is effective with Loosening Meditation. A client becomes expressive, feeling more confidence by practicing with music and sound. Music is effective for a patient with terminal illness to alleviate doubt, anger and fear and to come to a sense of acceptance with their lives in their remaining time, better preparing to pass on.

Using music during meditation can surely change and individual's

に瞑想を実施することは、介護で疲れている家族への支援としても有効です。

4) 臨床瞑想法に役立つ音楽の利用など

　臨床瞑想法に音楽を取り入れるのも効果的です。環境音楽のような静かな音やナレーションをCDやDVDを使って流すことで、瞑想の導入がスムーズになります。私は音楽療法士（岐阜県音楽療法士協会認定）として、お寺や病院、現在は東北地方の被災地でも、音楽療法と瞑想療法を併用した実践を行ってきました。

　お寺には多くの鳴り物があり、飛騨千光寺での臨床瞑想法の研修では、チベッタンベルや鈴、シンギングベル、リン、大鐘などいろいろ使っています。がん末期や慢性疾患の方々に、好みを聞いたうえで音楽を選択し、BGMのように音や音楽を流しながら臨床瞑想法を実践し、有意味な時間を提供した臨床事例があります。

　瞑想中のイメージを手助けし、回想する瞑想に役立てていますが、ゆるめる瞑想には特に効果的です。音や音楽を活用することは、その人の内的な感情表現を高め、自信を感じさせたり、末期患者であれば心の中の疑いや怒り、恐れをなだめ、人生の最期に残された時間の生き方、死に方など、心の整理をする手段を与えたりする効果があります。

　瞑想の中で音楽を活用することは、スピリチュアリティの変容に大きな影響を与えます。「音楽イメージ誘導法」(Guided Imagery and Music；GIM)では、クライアントの好む音楽や心理的に有効な音楽を活用して、イメージを誘発もしくはガイドし、ポジティブな意識状態をつくり出すことにあります。

　つまり音楽を用いてスピリチュアリティを変容させ、苦痛の緩和や生き方の再構築を目指します。このセラピーも、トランスパーソナル心理学などに基づいて研究されてきたものです。したがって、セラピストはある程度、近代の心理学や心理療法を常に学んでいることが、実践への手助けともなります。

　瞑想では自己意識の洞察が行われますが、音楽を流すことでより早く深い

experience with spirituality. A client's favorite music or psychologically effective music induces and guides positive imagery during "Guided imagery and Music". That is, the aims of using music are enhancing spiritual experience, alleviating pain and helping patients adjust their views of life if the client so desires. This therapy is explored within aspects of transpersonal psychology. Therefore, learning modern psychology and psychotherapy is helpful for leaders of Clinical mediation if they are not already trained as therapists.

A client can attain deeper insight into their consciousness by using music during meditation.

There are three basic ways to use music during meditation.

① Using music from beginning to end of meditation.

② Using music during the introductory parts of meditation.

③ Using music when finishing the meditation to cool down.

Please try the different ways above in exploring which way is most useful to you in leading meditation in accordance with the preferences of various clients. You should understand that using music is not always recommended because it sometimes also disturbs the mind. In some cases, it is useful for clients not to use music. I recommend using calm and relaxed music during the introductory part of breathing as it becomes easier to enter a meditative state.

5) The keys for practicing Clinical Meditation

To summarize, here are the main keys to Clinical Meditation:

① When you practice Clinical Meditation, you sit in the chair near the patient's bed and explain the meditation. You must not ever pressure them into meditating. Obtain the patient's consent and carefully explain how meditation can have an effect on making the heart feeling

境地に達することができるのです。

　瞑想時に音楽を活用する際には、次の3つの方法があります。

①はじめから最後まで音楽をかける。

②導入部分だけ音楽を活用する。

③終了時のクールダウンにだけ音楽を活用する。

　　どれが自分のリードに有効か、相手もあることですからいろいろ試してみてください。音楽によって、感情が乱れることもありますから万能ではないことも知ってください。対象者によっては、音楽を使わない瞑想法が有用なこともあります。

　　ちなみに、心が安らかになる音楽であれば、最初の呼吸法のところで流すのがおすすめです。スムーズに瞑想に入ることができます。

5）臨床瞑想法実践のポイント

　臨床現場で瞑想を指導（リード）するうえでのポイントを再掲します。実践を深めるために、繰り返し確認してください。

①臨床瞑想法を実施するときは、仰臥位のクライアントのベッドサイドに自分も腰を下ろし、説明を行います。瞑想が心を軽くする効果があることについて、十分に理解されるよう話し、同意を得ることが大切です。決して強制や圧力にならないようにご注意ください。

②入院施設で臨床瞑想法を実施するときは、まずクライアントが身体の不調や違和感がないかなどを確認してください。特に身体の痛みや微妙な違和感は意識の集中を妨げますので、期待する瞑想効果が得られない可能性があります。身体に関する不調和は、医療スタッフと相談し、疼痛コントロールのケアを施してから瞑想を導入してください。

③瞑想が禁忌（適用できない状態）とされるものとして、精神病、重症のうつ、急性錯乱状態、極度の不安、認知症などが含まれていますので、クライアントの症状を見極める慎重さは不可欠です。懸念される場合は、専門家に

light.

② When you practice Clinical Meditation in a hospital, the client's level of physical comfort or discomfort is confirmed. Pain or other subtle disorders in the body often disturbs a client's concentration. As a result, the client may not obtain the state they hope for. Please introduce meditation after relieving pain in consultation with medical staff.

③ Mental conditions, major depression, acute confused states, extreme anxiety and dementia are contraindication of meditation. You should prudently see the condition of a client. When you have any concerns, you consult a professional before you make a decision to practice meditation with the client.

④ Especially, prior to Watching meditation and Insight meditation, which involve the client's unconscious mind, you must make sure you have an understanding of the client's condition. Various emotions may arise and be unsettled in the client. If you are unable to confirm the meditation will be safe with them, you should consult with another expert for support. Don't feel pressure to solve it by your own efforts alone. Prioritize ethical and legal standards for your position and workplace when making such decisions.

⑤ Unconscious issues (e.g., trauma, PTSD) buried deep in a client's mind sometimes arise during meditation. This can lead them to states of temporary excitement or occasional incontinence. You as a therapist should be aware that such cases are not abnormal. For example, when a client cries bitterly, you make every effort to comfort them as permissible to your role and facility/workplace regulations. Such acute reactions of the client may be caused by separation anxiety in childhood or other previous life events. In such cases, meditation sessions may need to be combined with grief care, trauma care, or other forms of

相談の上で実施してください。

④具体的な観察瞑想や洞察瞑想を行う際には、特に注意が必要です。クライアントの、普段は意識化していない心に関与していきますので、いろいろな感情や振れが生じてきます。それを受け止めるあなたであってほしいと思いますが、もし「私は受け止められない」と判断したら、専門家（スピリチュアルケア専門職や心理カウンセリンセラーなど）に応援を依頼し、決して１人で抱え込まないでください。ただ、クライアントの「今ここで解決したい」とか「今のこの心をわかってほしい」という時間的制約のある場合は、そこでいったん受け止めてみる経験も大事です。

⑤臨床瞑想法を実施する課程で、クライアント自身が心の奥に封印していた課題（トラウマ、PTSDなど）が、表出することがあります。それによって、一時的に興奮したり、感情失禁したりするような事態が起こることもあります。しかし、セラピストはそういう現象は当たり前と受け止めて、冷静な行動をとってください。つまり、大泣きするというようなときは、本人の了解を得て、そっと肩や背中に手をあて、幼児を撫でるように温かく接してください。多くは幼児期の分離不安や、過去の悲しい出来事が関係していることが多く、その方のグリーフケアにかかわることも少なくありません。

心のケアや対人援助をする人は、日ごろから自身のことを相談できるスーパーバイザーとなる人を持つことが重要かと思います。そしていつでも困ったときに、相談できるゆとりが欲しいものです。

care.

Those who provide mental health care and collaborative services should have a supervisor with whom they usually consult with about their own concerns and should have mental space to consult whenever they are concerned about something.

> 第5章

臨床瞑想法指導者養成研修会の様子

　臨床瞑想法教育研究所では、飛騨千光寺境内にある国際平和瞑想センターを利用して、年間に10回ほどの「臨床瞑想法指導者養成研修会」が行われています。

　当研究所では、臨床瞑想法を取得し、実践できる養成講習会を開催しております。

【コース】

　①基礎編、②上級編、③指導編（各12時間、1泊2日）があり、千光寺の他、東京、名古屋、神戸などでも開講しています。

【認定証】

　合計36時間の過程を終了すると「臨床瞑想法指導者講習会終了証」を「臨床瞑想法教育研究所」から授与されます。

【研修の目的】

①自身のための瞑想法を習得できる。

②自身やケアの場面における生死観を考えることができる

③自身やケアに役立てるスピリチュアルケアを学ぶことができる

④自己を観察・洞察して内面的な世界観を広げることができる

⑤他者に対する臨床瞑想の指導法を習得することができる

【講習内容】

　「個人のスキルアップのための瞑想法」と「臨床現場で応用実践できる瞑

Section 5.

Certificate program for leaders of Clinical Meditation

The Clinical Meditation Research Institute, has an education course to train leaders of Clinical Meditation ten times per year at the International Peace Meditation Center, located in Hida-Senkōji Temple.

You can learn and practice Clinical Meditation by participating in sessions there, though up to now all sessions have been in Japanese.

【Courses】
Training is separated into three sections: ① Basic course, ②Advanced course, ③ Clinical Meditation Leader course (for twelve hours each over the course of two days). We have sessions at Hida-Senkōji, and at sites in Tokyo, Nagoya, Kobe and other sites around Japan.

【Certification】
Those who complete all three above courses can receive a certificate of completion in leading Clinical Meditation.

【The goals of these sessions】
① To learn Clinical Meditation for yourself.
② To reflect more deeply on your own views of life and death related to care of yourself and others.
③ To learn spiritual care for helping yourself and others.
④ To broaden your inner worldview through deepening observation of

想法」を３段階で習得できます。

　１回目）基礎編　12時間
　　臨床瞑想法の「ゆるめる瞑想法」「みつめる瞑想法」の基礎理論と基礎
　　実習
　２回目）上級編　12時間
　　臨床瞑想法の「たかめる瞑想法」「ゆだねる瞑想法」の発展理論と実習
　３回目）指導編　12時間
　　臨床瞑想法指導法の理論と実習　（集団指導法、個人指導法）

【研修会場】〜飛騨千光寺の紹介

　海抜約 900 メートルの山中に広がる境内には、大慈門の近くに「円空仏寺宝館」があり、館内には 64 体の円空仏と寺宝の一部が展示されています。さらに、本堂や庫裡などがある境内中心地を囲むように、山中に整備された八十八ヵ所の遍路道には、樹齢 1200 年を超える五本杉（国指定天然記念物）や愛宕社鎮守堂などの信仰の場所が点在し、山全体が信仰の対象となっています。

　町の喧噪も、鬱蒼とした緑に遮られ、聞こえるのは、ただ風の音と小鳥のさえずりのみ。ここではまるで時間が止まったかのように静寂があたりを支配します。

　また自然の散策を楽しむ八十八ヶ所霊場巡りは、当寺を囲む森の中に設けられた約３時間の徒歩コースです。

【注・資料】

１）A:（日本学術振興会 NO：21K07344「軽度認知障害者（MCI）および軽度認知症を（PwD）を対象としたゆるめる瞑想の効果〜瞑想セッション前後の心身の健康感と認知機能を調査する前向き観察研究〜 2022 」

　Effectiveness of Meditation to Rescue All people with Dementia and mild cognitive impairment (EMERALD) study by Dr.Hironisi, Dr.Kajimoto, Ven.

your heart and mind.

⑤To learn the method of guiding Clinical Meditation for others.

【Contents of the certification courses】

You learn and increase your skill in meditation and "Practical approach to Clinical Meditation in Medical Settings" in three steps.

① Basic course: 12 hours

Learn the basic theory and practice of "Loosening Meditation" and "Observing Meditation."

② Advanced course: 12 hours

Learn the advanced theory and practice of "Energizing Meditation" and "Unifying Meditation."

③ Clinical Meditation Leadership course: 12 hours

Learn the theory and practice of the methods of instruction for Clinical Meditation to guide it for both individuals and groups.

【Venue of the Certificate Training sessions ～ What is it like at Hida-Senkōji Temple?】

Clinical Meditation Education Institute/International Peace Meditation Center

Senkōji Temple

Nyukawa, Takayama, Gifu, Japan   zip 506-2135

Tel: 0577-78-1021

http://senkouji.com/   https://www.rinmeiso.com

◉An Ancient Temple Founded Over 1,600 Years Ago

Senkōji Temple is said to have been founded as a place of prayer 1,600

Oshita et al.

B:「山本明弘「軽度認知機能障害または認知症者の介護家族に対する『ゆるめる瞑想』の精神的健康、心理的ストレス反応および介護負担の変化を調査する前向き観察研究」（2023、日本スピリチュアルケア学会）に発表。調査には、精神的健康の評価は GHQ（General Health Questionnaire）30 項目を、心理的ストレス反応の評価は SRS（Stress Response Scale）18 項目を、介護負担の評価は日本版 ZBI（Zarit Caregiver Burden Interview）8 項目を用いた。結果は、介護家族が「ゆるめる瞑想会」に参加することによって、3 指標ともに第 1 回直前と比較して第 1 回直後に有意な低下を示した。また GHQ30 では、第 4 回直後および第 4 回 2 週間後でも有意な低下を示した。ゆるめる瞑想には介護家族の精神的健康増進、ストレスおよび介護負担緩和効果のあることが示唆された。

2）日本成人病予防協会 HP（japa.org）の報告では、ストレスを無くす努力をするよりも、いかに「悪いストレスを良いストレスに変えていくか」が重要と説明する。例えば、書類の提出期限を目標と捉えてバネにしてがんばる人もいますが、迫り来る締切と感じて自分を苦しめる人もいる。「ストレス」を乗り越えて得られる「快感」は、「達成感」、「満足感」となる。ストレスの概念を医学界に取り入れたセリエ博士は、ストレスは人生のスパイスと表現している。

3）健康生成（Salutogenesis）はラテン語のサルス（salus: 健康）とギリシャ語のジェネス（genesis: 生成）からなる概念で、個人が健康を増進するうえで助けとなる力についてのこと。近年ではレジリエンス（resilience）の概念や、アントノフスキー（Aaron Antonovsky、1987）のセンス・オブ・コヒアランス（Sense of Coherence ＝ SOC）: 首尾一貫感覚などが健康生成論の中心的概念となっている。

4）トランスパーソナル心理学は（Transpersonal psychology）人間性心理学を発展させ、ヒューマンポテンシャル運動・ニューエイジの人間観を取り入れた心理学で、個体的・個人的（パーソナル）なものを超える（トランス）、または通り抜けることを目指し、あるいはそうした経験を重視する。トランスパーソナルな経験、通常の人間個人の限りある自己意識が拡大し、より大きな、より意味に満ちた現実とつながる経験や、死後の世界や宇宙空間、母胎への回帰や過去生のイメージ体験等を重視する。

years ago by Ryomen Sukuna, the prominent Hida clan leader during the reign of Emperor Nintoku. It was officially established as a Buddhist temple 400 years later when Prince Shinnyo, a son of Emperor Saga and one of the ten great disciples of Kukai (Kobo Daishi), built a Shingon esoteric Buddhist prayer hall in Hida. At its peak, it boasted nineteen temples and monastic quarters on the mountainside, all of which were destroyed by fire when the Takeda army of Kai attacked Hida in Eiroku 7 (1564).

At an elevation of approximately 900 meters, Senkōji Temple sits near the peak of Mount Kesa, where silence prevails. Nestled amidst lush foliage, the temple finds solace away from the bustling town below, where only the soft whispers of the wind and the melodious chirping of birds break the silence. It's as if time itself has paused in this serene environment.

Visitors have the opportunity to enjoy nature walks around the Eighty-Eight Sacred Sites, following a roughly three-hour walking course through the forest surrounding the temple.

Beyond its religious practices, Senkōji Temple has established the International Peace Meditation Center, offering various meditation-focused training programs, such as the Clinical Meditation Method, for healing and self-discovery. In addition to medical care, welfare, and education, programs are available for corporate training, including perspectives on life and death, spiritual care, meditation sessions, and relaxation.

【Notes】

1) A: Hironishi M, Kajimoto Y, Oshita D. (2022). *Effectiveness of meditation to rescue all people with dementia and mild cognitive impairment (EMERALD study).* Japan Society for Promotion of Science.

B: Yamamoto A. (2023). *Effects of Loosening meditation on mental health, psychological stress and burden for caregivers who care for patients with mild cognitive impairment and dementia: prospective study (tentative title).* Annual

（村川治彦「アメリカにおけるニューエイジ運動の源流とその特徴（前半）」（PDF）
『ホリスティック教育研究』第 7 巻、日本ホリスティック教育協会、2004 ほか）

5）シャマタ瞑想について、仏教経典の『入出息念経』（ānāpānasati-Sutta）では、
森や樹木の下、あるいは室内などで、出入りの呼吸に注意を凝らし、「身体のス
キャン（身体）し、その感覚を感じ（感受）、そして心の状態を観察し（観心）、
やがてその心を拡大しつつ、あらゆる執着を手放して、平安で静寂なこころに
到達する（観法）」修習法である、と説明されている。

6）唯識論とは玄奘三蔵の説いたもので、玄奘三蔵は中国からインドまで往復し
て仏典を持ち帰った人として有名である。（唯識学会 HP より）

（a）唯識は 仏教の人間学であり、人間とは何か？ を説いた心理学ともいえる。

（b）唯識学は、信じることよりまず理解することを教える。（c）唯識は、現実の自
分を、立ち止まって凝視することから始まる。現実の自分とは、自分の根底（無）
の部分を含む存在の全体の働きを自覚することである。（d）スイスの精神医学者
ユングは、「自分の体験するものはすべて心的現象にある。人間の心という永遠
の事実の上に自分の基礎を築くために、自分という主観的存在（本当の無の自分）
の、もっと独自にして内奥の基礎を知り、これを認識したい」という思いから、
精神医学を始めた。（e）仏陀のいう「自らを灯とし帰依処とせよ」とは、本来の
自分を見つめ、それをよりどころとしなさい、ということ。

　この他に、仏教用語が出てくる文章があります。本書での解説には限りがある
ために、興味のある方は仏教辞典や専門書を参照ください。

【謝辞】

　本書の製作には下記の方が編集に協力してくださいましたことに感謝しま
す。編者の多くは、臨床瞑想法教育研究所が主催する「臨床瞑想法指導者養
成講習会」を受講修了された方々で、自身の体験からも編集にご協力いただ
きました。とくに初版の翻訳には宮本圭子さんの尽力があったことを心より
感謝と御礼を申し上げます。

Meeting of Japan Society for Spiritual Care.

In this study, mental health was assessed by a General Health Questionnaire (GHQ) consisting of 30 items, psychological stress by Stress Response Scale (SRS) consisting of 18 items and burden of care by Zarit Caregiver Burden Interviews Japanese ver. (ZBI) consisting of 8 items. The results show that all three scores after the first stage of meditation were significantly better than before the first stage of meditation. And GHQ scores significantly improved after the fourth stage of meditation and four weeks later, more improvement than before the fourth. The results suggested that Loosening Meditation had an effect on improving mental health, relieving stress and lowering the burden of care in caregivers.

2) Japan Preventive Association for Adult Diseases explains that it is more important to change bad stress to good stress rather than making an effort of getting rid of stress. For example, some people are driven by a deadline as a goal. When they can meet the deadline, they have satisfaction and fulfilment by overcoming stress. While, others are depressed by being overwhelmed by the deadline.

3) Salutogenesis is a coined word consisted of "salus (health)" in Latin and "genese (generation)" in Greek and means the power to help improve health. Recently, the theory of resilience and Sense of Coherence (SOC) by Antonovsky (1987) is the central concept of salutogenesis.

4) Transpersonal psychology developed from humanistic psychology and was adopted in the Human Potential Movement and perspectives of the New Age Movement. Murakawa H. (2004). The origin and the characteristics of the New Age movement in US (the first half). *Study in Holistic Education (7)*. (In Japanese).

5) Nyū shutsusoku nenkyō (Anapanasati Sutta 入出息念経) in Buddhist doctrine explains that Shamata meditation is the method of practice of scanning the body, observing sensations in one's body, observing the mind, and attaining

●**編集者**（敬称略）

大下大圓（臨床瞑想法教育研究所代表、飛騨千光寺長老、和歌山県立医科大学連携教授）　daien@senkouji.com　：vazara@senkouji.com

宮本圭子（大阪大学産業科学研究所技術補佐員・一般社団法人テラプロジェクト研究員）

西垣悦代（関西医科大学医学部心理学教室教授）

齊藤弘久（東京大学大学院総合文化研究科附属国際交流センター特任准教授）

ミション・ネイサン慈心（龍谷大学非常勤教授、インワードジャーニージャパン代表）

ノーブル慧光（アメリカ在住、元大学教員、真言宗僧侶）

a peaceful and calm state, deepening spirituality and releasing attachments while focusing on breathing meditation, out-of- doors in a forest under trees or indoors in the meditation hall or other place of practice.

6) Yuishiki (唯識) means subconscious mind which consists of five senses and sixth sense of consciousness (Sonen 想念), Manashiki 末那識 and Arayashiki 阿頼耶識 in Buddhist psychology. Reportedly, Genjō Sanzō (玄奘三蔵) a famous monk in the 7th century brought Buddhist scriptures from India to China and first transmitted the Yuishiki teachings and philosophy.

(a) Yuishiki (vijñapti-mātratā) is anthropology in Buddhism. It is a psychology which explains what a human being is.

(b) The theory of Yuishiki teaches that understanding is more important than believing.

(c) Yuishiki starts from stopping and penetrating oneself. Knowing one's true self is conscious of all of functions including basic and unconscious being.

(d) Jung was a Swiss psychiatrist who thought that all experiences were psychic phenomena. He hoped to know and admit original and inner subjective existence to build his foundation on human psychology as external facts. Those thoughts inspired him to start studying psychiatry.

(e) Making one's self a source of light and believing it as Buddha's word means observing one's true self and the base of one's thought.: 唯識とは | 唯識学会 (yuishiki.org)

For more in depth explanation of many Buddhist terms in this text, an excellent online resource in English is the Digital Dictionary of Buddhism (http://buddhism-dict.net/ddb/index.html, password: guest), and other reference works are available.

【Afterword】

I appreciate the support of members of the Editorial Board who

contributed to this book. Most all are engaged in the Leadership Training Course offered at the Clinical Meditation Education Research Institute. Their participation in editing this book is based on their experience in meditation. I offer special thanks to Keiko Miyamoto who translated the first edition into English.

● Editorial Board

Rev. Maha-Acharyā, Daien Oshita (大下大圓, 伝燈大阿闍梨): Hida-Senkōji Elder, Director, Clinical Meditation Education Research Institute/ International Peace Meditation Center, Wakayama Medical University, Associate Professor. daien@senkouji.com

Ms. Keiko Miyamoto: Laboratory assistant, Sanken, Institute of Scientific and Industrial Research, Osaka University, Researcher at the Thera-Project, MPH

Dr. Etsuyo Nishigaki (西垣悦代): Professor of Psychology, Kansai Medical University, Osaka, Japan

Dr. Hirohisa Saitō (齋藤弘久): Specially Appointed Associate Professor, Graduate School of Arts and Sciences, International Exchange Center, Tokyo University, Tokyo, Japan

Rev. Dr. Nathan Jishin Michon (ネイサン・慈心・ミション): Ryukoku University; Director, Inward Journeys Japan

Rev. Acharyā Ekō Noble (ノーブ・慧光, 阿闍梨): Founder and Spiritual Director, Radiant Light Sangha, Portland, Oregon, USA

●編著者略歴

大下大圓（おおした・だいえん）

飛騨千光寺長老、国際平和瞑想センター代表、和歌山県立医科大学連携教授、沖縄大学客員教授、名古屋大学医学部非常勤講師、高野山伝燈阿闍梨。12歳で出家得度、高野山で修行、阿闍梨となる。高野山大学仏教学科卒。岐阜大学教育学部研究生、京都大学こころの未来研究センターで瞑想の臨床応用を研究し、臨床瞑想法のメソッドを開発。京都大学など医学、看護学、教育学、福祉学の大学で死生学、スピリチュアルケア学などの非常勤講師をつとめ、現在は、日本ホスピス在宅ケア研究会理事、日本スピリチュアルケア学会理事、NPO法人日本スピリチュアルケアワーカー協会副会長、日本臨床宗教師会副会長などをつとめる。著書に『臨床瞑想法』、『実践的スピリチュアルケア』、『密教 大楽に生きるワザ』、『講座スピリチュアル学 第1巻 スピリチュアルケア』（共著）『ACP 人生会議でこころのケア』（共著）ほか多数。

臨床瞑想法のためのメソッド紹介
その魅力と実践法

2025年2月26日 初版第1刷発行

著　者　　大下大圓
発行者　　埋田喜子
発行所　　株式会社 ビイング・ネット・プレス
〒252-0303 神奈川県相模原市南区相模大野 8-2-12-202
電話 042（702）9213
デザイン　山田孝之
印　刷　　モリモト印刷株式会社

ISBN 978-4-908055-34-8 C0011
printed in japan
© 2025 by Oshita Daien

memo

memo